The Economics of Medical Care: A Policy Perspective

Joseph P. Newhouse
The Rand Corporation

ADDISON-WESLEY PUBLISHING COMPANY
Reading, Massachusetts • Menlo Park, California
London • Amsterdam • Don Mills, Ontario • Sydney

ISBN 0-201-08369-8
ABCDEFGHIJK-AL-798

The Economics of
Medical Care:
A Policy Perspective

PERSPECTIVES ON ECONOMICS SERIES

Michael L. Wachter & Susan M. Wachter, Editors

PUBLISHED

**Development, The International Economic Order
and Commodity Agreements,** *Jere R. Behrman*
**The Economics of Medical Care:
A Policy Perspective,** *Joseph P. Newhouse*
Money and Economy: A Monetarist View, *William Poole*
Antitrust Policies and Issues, *Roger Sherman*
Income Distribution and Redistribution, *Paul J. Taubman*

AVAILABLE IN LATE 1978 AND EARLY 1979

Labor Unions, *George H. Hildebrand*
Forecasting, *Lawrence R. Klein & Richard M. Young*
International Trade, *Stephen P. Magee*
Regulation, *Roger G. Noll*
Population, *T. Paul Schultz*
Urban Economics, *Susan M. Wachter*

Foreword

The PERSPECTIVES ON ECONOMICS series has been developed to present economics students with up-to-date policy-oriented books written by leading scholars in this field. Many professors and students have stressed the need for flexible, contemporary materials that provide an understanding of current policy issues.

In general, beginning students in economics are not exposed to the controversial material and development of current issues that are the basis of research in economics. Because of their length and breadth of coverage, textbooks tend to lack current economic thinking on policy questions; in attempting to provide a balanced viewpoint, they often do not give the reader a feel for the lively controversy in each field. With this series, we have attempted to fill this void.

The books in this series are designed to complement standard textbooks. Each volume reflects the research interests and views of the authors. Thus these books can also serve as basic reading material in the specific topic courses covered by each. The stress throughout is on the careful development of institutional factors and policy in the context of economic theory. Yet the exposition is designed to be accessible to undergraduate students and interested laypersons with an elementary background in economics.

Michael L. Wachter
Susan M. Wachter

Preface

This book illustrates the application of microeconomic theory to the economics of medical care. It should, therefore, aid the student in understanding economic theory as well as the economics of medical care.

Medical care has become increasingly significant in our nation's economy. It now makes up nearly 9 percent of our Gross National Product, and is a major topic of public policy. All levels of government are involved in its financing and regulation. There is widespread controversy about what kinds of new legislation are required, especially at the federal level. Unfortunately, the economics literature that might illuminate the debate is sparse.

This book is designed to supplement the basic text in an introductory microeconomics course, as well as for an upper-level undergraduate course on the economics of health or medical care, or for courses in medical schools and schools of public health dealing with the subject. Health professionals who have had no prior exposure to economics will probably find some of the material explained too tersely. If so, they should read selected chapters of an introductory economics textbook. Introductory chapters covering demand or theory of the consumer are relevant to Chapter 2 in this book; the chapters covering production and supply or theory of the firm are relevant to Chapter 3; the chapters covering the operation of markets, especially competitive markets, are relevant to Chapter 4; and the chapters on welfare economics, government intervention, and market failure are relevant to Chapter 6.

The author would like to thank Robert Brook, William Schwartz, Kathleen Williams, and Mark Pauly for helpful comments on an earlier draft. Their advice was not always heeded, and so they cannot be held responsible for the contents.

May 1978   J. P. N.
Santa Monica, California

Contents

INTRODUCTION   **1**
    References   **3**

**THE DEMAND FOR MEDICAL CARE SERVICES AND THE
DEMAND FOR HEALTH INSURANCE**   **4**
    The Theory of the Demand for Medical Care   5
    Empirical Evidence   15
    The Demand for Insurance   19
    References   23

PHYSICIAN SUPPLY   **25**
    The Federal Government and Medical Schools   25
    Financing Medical Schools   26
    The Capacity of Medical Schools   32
    Studies Made by Previous Manpower Planners   43
    References   47

THE MEDICAL MARKETPLACE   **49**
    Do Physicians Maximize Profits?   50
    What are the Consequences of Restricting Entry?   53
    Consumer Ignorance   54
    Do Physicians Create Their Own Demand?   55
    What is the Basis for Price Competition in an Insured Market?   61
    Conclusion   65
    References   66

APPENDIX TO CHAPTER 4: HOW DO HOSPITALS MAKE
    CHOICES   68

Do Hospitals Minimize Costs?   69
Choosing the Wrong Products   70
Does Divergence from Perfect Competition Really Represent Inefficiency?   71
References   72

THE OUTPUT OF THE MEDICAL CARE DELIVERY SYSTEM   74

References   87

PLAN AND MARKET ALTERNATIVES TO THE STATUS QUO:
    TECHNIQUES FOR MANAGING RESOURCE ALLOCA-
    TION IN MEDICAL CARE   89

The Properties of Perfectly Competitive Markets   89
Problems Connected with Organizing the Medical Care Sector to
    Resemble a Perfectly Competitive Market   95
Regulation or Planning of Medical Services   100
Changing Medical Care Institutions to More Closely Resemble a
    Competitive Market   108
References   113
INDEX   115

Introduction   1

This book discusses the economics of medical care. Why is this topic important? First, medical care is an important part of our economy. Currently, more than one-twelfth of measured economic activity is in medical care (8.6 percent of Gross National Product in fiscal 1976 [1]), and this percentage has been rapidly growing in recent years (see Table 1.1). Reflecting this growth, the number of employees in medical care has also grown rapidly—5.4 percent of those employed in 1974 worked in medical care.

Table 1.1 Medical care expenditure and employment, selected years

Year	Expenditure as percentage of GNP*	Employment as percentage of employed persons†
1929	3.5	—
1940	4.1	—
1950	4.5	3.0
1960	5.2	4.0
1970	7.2	4.0
1974	7.8	5.4†
1976	8.6	—

*Fiscal years. (*Source:* Robert M. Gibson and Marjorie S. Mueller, "National Health Expenditures, Fiscal Year 1976," *Social Security Bulletin* 40: Table 1 (April 1977).

†1950, 1960, and 1970 figures from Decennial Census. Reported in United States Public Health Service, "Health Manpower Source Book, Section 17," 1963, Tables 1, 6, and p. 12, and United States Public Health Service, "Health Resources Statistics: 1975," Table 2. The 1974 figure is also from "Health Resources Statistics: 1975," Table 1, but may not be comparable to the other figures because it is based largely on reports of professional associations, whereas the census figures are based on individual respondents. Total civilian employment in 1974 is from *Economic Report of the President, 1977,* Table B-27.

Second, prices in medical care have been rising at above-average rates for many years, as shown in Table 1.2. As a result, when price controls were lifted from the rest of the economy in 1974, the Administration (unsuccessfully) proposed to keep them applicable to medical care. In 1977, a new Administration sought legislative authority to control medical care costs. In this book we will examine why prices have been rising so rapidly and provide a basis for appraising the public debate over controlling medical care costs.

Table 1.2 Medical care price increases compared to all goods

Years	Average percentage rate of increase	
	Medical care	All items
1940–1950	3.9	5.6
1950–1960	3.9	2.1
1960–1970	4.3	2.7
1970–1976	7.4	6.6
1950–1976	4.9	3.4

Source: *Economic Report of the President, 1977,* Table B–47. 1976 value is for July.

Third, medical care is now and will almost certainly remain a major public policy issue. Forty-two percent of all medical care expenditures now come from the public treasury (up from 26 percent in 1950), and numerous regulations and laws apply to the medical care sector and affect how it functions. Countless new proposals are offered each year at the federal, state, and local levels to change public policy toward medical care. An important proposal is that of establishing a national health insurance plan. Unlike earlier eras, when political debate swirled around the question of whether there should be a national health insurance plan at all [2,3], today's debate concerns what kind of national health insurance plan there should be. As will be seen, economic analysis provides a framework for understanding the issues involved in this debate.

Fourth, analysis of medical care economics should help you learn microeconomic theory, for it will illustrate several important economic principles. By studying an example of how economic theory can be applied, you may achieve a better understanding of economic principles and how they may be used to analyze areas of human activity.

Finally, medical care is important to people's well-being. Many believe medical care is so important that it should be readily available without charge to all. Reality dictates compromise with this position; for example, some services will never be located in rural areas. Nonetheless, the prevalence of this view underlines the social significance of medical care, especially when one reflects that hardly anyone argues that food or clothing should be universally available without charge. The economic organization of medical care and its cost affects the health and well-being of the population by determining *who* is treated, *for what* type of medical problem, *by whom* the treatment is given, *how* the person is treated, and *how much* the person giving the treatment is paid.

Defining medical care services is an important preliminary matter. I include as medical care services: hospital care, services of physicians, dentists, and other health professionals, drugs, eyeglasses, medical supplies (such as bandages), and nursing home care. I have chosen not to analyze traditional government public health activities such as ensuring a clean water supply or the purity of food served in restaurants. Financing these activities is less controversial than financing many of the personal medical care services discussed below. Moreover, analyzing public health activities requires an exposition of the theory of public goods.

The plan of the book is as follows. In the next chapter we will analyze the demand for medical care services and its relationship to health insurance. As will quickly become apparent, insurance plays a critical role in the economics of medical care. Then we consider two topics in the supply of medical care services: how medical schools are financed and the number of physicians that medical schools should train. This chapter may be of special interest to premedical or medical students. Then we will look at the operation of the medical marketplace, where suppliers and demanders meet. Whereas the previous two chapters focused on decisions of individuals and firms, this chapter looks at the results of those decisions in the medical marketplace. An appendix to Chapter 4 contains a discussion of the special economics of the nonprofit hospital. In Chapter 5 we take up the issue of what might be expected from further investment in medical care services; given that various national health insurance plans may well expand the quantity of resources in medical care, what can the nation expect to obtain in return? The concluding chapter considers the question of reform in the medical care marketplace, in particular the role for regulation and the possibilities for increased price competition.

REFERENCES

1. Robert M. Gibson and Marjorie S. Mueller. "National Health Expenditures, Fiscal Year 1976," *Social Security Bulletin* 40, No. 4: 3–22 (April 1977).

2. Theodore R. Marmor. *The Politics of Medicare*. Chicago, Ill.: Aldine, 1973.

3. Richard Harris. *A Sacred Trust*. Baltimore, Md.: Penguin, 1969.

The Demand for 2
Medical Care Services
and the Demand for
Health Insurance

We begin our look at the economics of medical care by studying the important concept of demand. The quantity of medical care demanded is how many services individuals (or physicians acting as their agents) *seek to* purchase; when combined with the quantity of services supplied or available, the quantity demanded determines actual utilization. The quantity demanded may be sufficiently large that some demand is unsatisfied. In this event, the medical care delivery system will appear stressed. The amount of stress will affect such phenomena as prices, waiting times for an appointment, and perhaps the amount of time physicians spend with patients.

In addition to determining the amount of stress on the delivery system, the study of demand is important for at least two other reasons. Health financing is a major public policy issue, and it is important to know how different subgroups of the population—for example, the poor—will react to different financing arrangements. Second, how different insurance arrangements affect demand helps determine the desirable structure of health insurance. However, the relevance of demand to this issue will not be taken up until Chapter 6 (see p. 99).

In the subsequent chapters the demand for medical care plays a quite prominent role. A contrasting, possibly widely held view is that it is unimportant to study demand because when one is sick, one seeks or should seek medical care, and when one is well, one does not (save perhaps for an annual physical examination and immunizations). Moreover, according to this view, when one is sick there is a single method for treating one's illness; hence, demand is unimportant. This view underlies an important study in the 1930s [1] that was recently updated [2]. These studies employed the following methods. They estimated the amount of sickness in a given population, and then estimated the number of physicians "necessary" to treat that

4

amount of sickness. The 1930s study estimated that 135 physicians would be necessary for every 100,000 people. In other words, this technological view of medical care holds that the only important determinant of medical care demand is illness. As we shall show in this chapter, the evidence is not kind to this view. But before coming to the evidence, it is necessary to master some theory.

THE THEORY OF THE DEMAND FOR MEDICAL CARE

Let us assume that there are only two goods a consumer can buy, medical care and a composite commodity we shall call COMP. (We can allow COMP to consist of several commodities as long as their relative prices remain constant.) While this assumption of only two goods violates reality, it is essential if we are to employ graphical techniques rather than the calculus. Fortunately, the results we derive from this two-commodity world are equally applicable in a many-commodity world. We shall also assume that medical care and COMP are bought in units such that each unit of medical care costs P_M and each unit of COMP costs P_C. We then ask: How much medical care will be bought by a consumer who has an income of $\$I$ and spends that entire income?[1]

　　To solve this problem, we assume that the consumer has a utility function showing the amount of utility derived from varying amounts of medical care and COMP. For any given state of health, the consumer will accept more medical care and less COMP, or less medical care and more COMP, and feel equally well off. Combinations of medical care and COMP that leave the consumer equally well off lie along indifference curves; a set of indifference curves is shown in Fig. 2.1. If all income I is spent on medical care, M units of medical care will be consumed; if all income is spent on COMP, C units of COMP will be consumed. Given the prices of COMP and medical care, any combination of COMP and medical care that lies along the straight line that connects points M and C can be purchased. (Note that the line is straight because one more unit of medical care can always be bought by giving up P_M/P_C units of COMP, no matter how many units of medical care have already been purchased. Can you see why the trading ratio is 1 to P_M/P_C units?) The consumer's problem is to select the point along the straight line most preferred. The preferred point will be the one that places the consumer on the highest possible indifference curve; this point is W in Fig. 2.1. Thus, a consumer who acts as if a utility function is being maximized will buy the amount of medical care and COMP represented by point W in the figure.

---

1 The assumption that the consumer's entire income is spent also simplifies the exposition but is not critical to our results.

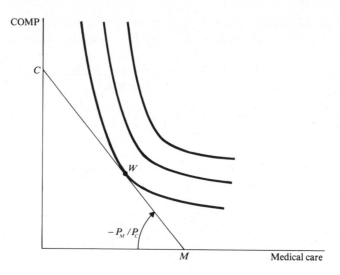

Fig. 2.1 Indifference curves and budget line to determine amount of medical care purchased: W is the highest attainable utility level, given the income represented by the line connecting C and M.

At this point you may think that the argument is too abstract, and that the last time you went to the doctor, the doctor prescribed a medical treatment that you instituted. Were you merely following the instructions of the doctor, so that it was meaningless to speak of deciding whether you wanted a little more COMP or a little more medical care (i.e., doing as the doctor advised)? Some individuals argue that economic theory does not apply to medical care because economic theory assumes a "rational, well-informed" consumer, and most consumers typically know relatively little about medical care.

Two types of responses may be offered to this objection. First, and most important, the proper test of a theory is how well it predicts real phenomena relative to other theories. Although we will not take account of other theories in this book, we will attempt to show that economic theory does give one considerable insight about medical care, and that it does predict a number of phenomena that are, in fact, observed.

Second, the theory outlined above requires only that *somebody* act in a maximizing (purposive) way. Although for most goods it is natural to think of the maximizer as the consumer, in medical care it may be more natural to think of the maximizer as some combination of the consumer and the physician. Clearly, a physician is critical to many choices in medical care. For example, a patient cannot be admitted to a hospital without a physician's approval, and certain drugs cannot be purchased without a physician's prescription. Yet it is equally clear that the consumer also plays a role. For example, the consumer generally makes the initial decision to seek care, and the vast literature on compliance indicates that patients do not always act in accordance with what a physician dictates.[2] Even more subtly, a physician may take account of a patient's economic circumstances when deciding on a course of treatment. In this sense, the physician acts as the patient's agent, ideally making those decisions that the patient would make if the patient knew as much about medicine as the physician. In such circumstances the outcome would be identical to that observed with perfectly informed consumers.

Enough of the digression concerning this objection. Let us exercise the model a bit. Suppose the price of medical care falls and that instead of costing P_M, medical care actually costs $P_M/2$, or one-half as much. How much medical care will then be consumed? As you may recall, a price change can be broken into a substitution and an income effect. These effects are diagrammed in Fig. 2.2. The new price line is represented by the line connecting C and $2M$. (Why is the point on the horizontal axis equal to $2M$?) At the new price, quantities of C and M given by the point X will be consumed. The substitution and the income effect come about because a fall in the price of a commodity, holding money income constant, not only makes that commodity relatively cheaper than other commodities, but also raises real income (that is, increases the total amount of goods and services that can be bought). Because the commodity is relatively cheaper, the consumer substitutes it for other commodities, and would do this even if the level of well-being (real income) were constant. This substitution effect is shown by the move from W to Y. Additionally, because the consumer's real income has risen, the consumer moves from point Y to point X. (Note that the dashed budget line through Y is parallel to the solid budget line through X, indicating that income has risen, while relative prices have remained unchanged between points X and Y.) Points W and X are two points on the demand curve of a consumer whose indifference curves are shaped like Fig. 2.2 and who has income $I. By drawing in price lines corresponding to prices other than P_M and $P_M/2$, we could find other points of tangency (in addition to W and X), and we could trace out a demand curve for medical care as its relative price varies. Such a demand curve is shown in Fig. 2.2b. It is drawn as a straight line, although the only restriction implied by the theory is that the line slopes from northwest to southeast.[3]

Now that we have diagrammed how demand for medical care changes in response to changes in its relative price, it is an easy step to understanding how health insurance affects demand. Suppose the consumer pays a certain

2 Compliance is whether a patient follows a physician's orders.

3 Assuming that as income rises (holding health status and other factors constant), demand for medical care does not fall.

insurance premium to purchase an insurance policy that covers 50 percent of the costs of medical care. Suppose that prior to purchasing the insurance policy the consumer's optimum was at point W in Fig. 2.2a. The insurance policy by definition reduces the price of medical care to the consumer to $P_M/2$. Does this mean the consumer will now consume X? The answer is no, because the premium payment must also be accounted for, and the premium reduces the consumer's income. Will this reduction in income move the consumer to a point where the consumer is less well off than at W (that is, on a lower indifference curve)? Presumably not if the consumer voluntarily bought the insurance, but if the insurance is in some way imposed on the consumer (for example, a law is enacted that each person must have a

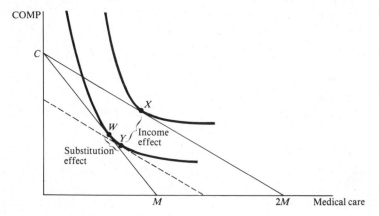

Fig. 2.2a A halving of the price of medical care. The consumer substitutes medical care for other commodities and is able to buy more of all commodities because real income has increased.

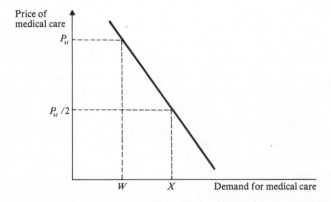

Fig. 2.2b A demand curve for medical care derived from the utility function and income level shown in Fig. 2.2a.

certain amount of health insurance), one needs more information before concluding that the insurance benefited or harmed the consumer. We shall return to judging the appropriate amount of insurance in Chapter 6 (see p. 99).

For the purpose of studying the relationship between health insurance and demand, the important point is that insurance is like a subsidy to purchase medical care; that is, it lowers the per-unit price of care. Although there is an income effect caused by the premiums or taxes paid to finance the insurance benefits, these income effects can be shown to be empirically negligible in their effect on the demand for care (although not necessarily on the level of utility!), and so it can be predicted that the more extensive the insurance (i.e., the lower the price to the consumer), the higher will be the demand for medical care. In other words, demand is not perfectly inelastic (the demand curve is not vertical).

Price elasticity is zero in a special case—the technological view of medical care referred to at the beginning of the chapter. This view emphasizes sickness, but sickness has not formally entered our model. It is time for sickness's entrance.

Any set of indifference curves is conditional upon a given state of health; if an individual's health changes, the indifference curves will change. Figure 2.3 shows how indifference curves may change if one be-

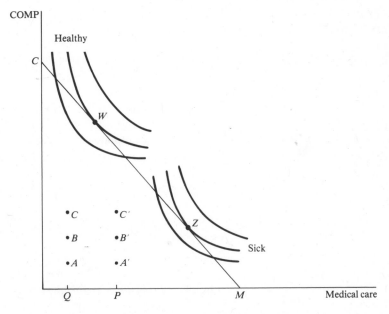

Fig. 2.3 How sickness changes the location of indifference curves.

comes sick. Suppose a healthy person with income as shown in the budget line in Fig. 2.3 will consume the quantities indicated by point W. If the person becomes sick, suppose the consumption bundle shifts to that represented by point Z. (Why does Z lie on the straight line connecting C and M?) The individual now spends more on medical care, and has less available to spend on COMP. Both in the figure and in real life, health status very much affects individual expenditure on medical care. But the technological view insists that *only* health status matters, clearly a much stronger statement than that health status is an important determinant of demand. How much stronger a statement can be seen by noting what happens to the indifference curves if only health status matters. With this assumption the "curves" become mere points that lie in a vertical line, such as points A, B, and C or A', B', and C' in Fig. 2.3. Given a level of illness, the individual consumes the amount Q of medical care (assuming income is sufficient to purchase an amount Q), irrespective of its price. If the illness is more severe, the individual consumes Q'. For a given level of illness the individual buys more COMP as income increases. Thus the technological view implies that expenditure on medical care is constant as income changes (assuming health unchanged), a conclusion clearly contradicted by the rising expenditure on medical care as GNP grows (Table 1.1), as well as data on consumption by individual households [3].

Because the indifference curve is a point, the technological view also implies that there are no substitutes for medical care; that is, the individual is not willing to trade some COMP for more medical care, or give up some medical care for more COMP (for example, not pay the dermatologist to prescribe a remedy for one's dandruff but use the money to buy a phonograph album instead).[4] As a result, the demand curve for medical care is perfectly inelastic and determined only by the patient's illness (some might say only by what the physician tells the patient about the illness).

A natural experiment that decisively rejects the technological view took place among employees of Stanford University and their dependents in 1966 and 1968 [4]. In 1966 the group had an insurance plan that completely covered physicians' services. Because the plan was running a deficit, the plan was altered so that individuals would pay one-fourth of the bill for physician services. The number of visits was recorded for those individuals who were in the plan in both 1966 and 1968. As compared with 1966, when services were free, there was a 25-percent drop in the number of physician visits in 1968, when the price jumped from zero to $P_M/4$. While it is possible that there was more sickness in 1966, it does not seem likely that sickness

---

4 The technological view also assumes that the *method* of treatment of a given problem is independent of all prices and income, but the weaknesses of that assumption cannot be dealt with here.

among a group of 2,567 people would vary sufficiently from one year to another to account for a 25-percent change in visits.

Other studies mentioned later in this chapter also conclude that demand does respond to changes in price, but before coming to them, we ask the further question: Do different groups in the population respond to changes in insurance differently? To place empirical data on this question in perspective, we need to develop a bit more theory.

Until now, we have been pretending that the only "price" the patient had to pay for a physician visit was a money price. In fact, there is another kind of price, a time price. All of us face the constraint that there are only twenty-four hours in a day. Some of those hours can be converted into money income by working. Let us assume that if one chooses to work an extra hour (or work an hour less), one's income would change by an amount equal to the hourly wage. Thus, if the individual uses an hour to visit the doctor instead of working (ignore sick-leave provisions for the moment), that person's income will fall by w, the hourly wage. It is just as though the price (to an uninsured person) of that hour's visit was $P_M + w$. In a more general case, health insurance may cover a certain fraction of the costs and visits may take more or less than one hour. Hence, we shall write the price of medical services as $cP_M + wt$, where c is the proportion of the price that is left to the patient to pay by an insurance plan (the coinsurance rate), and t is the time (in hours) that medical service takes. (What is c for the uninsured patient?) Note that the wage w is like a price of time for the individual.

With this formulation insight is available on how different groups are likely to react to change in insurance coverage. The smaller the time price (wt), the larger the percentage change in *total* price caused by a change in health insurance (i.e., in the parameter c). (You can see this by letting $P_M = 1$ and then considering the effect of changes in c if wt equals 1 and if wt equals 10. In the latter case, the total price of medical care is dominated by the time price.) Therefore, other factors equal, those individuals with *low* time prices will show a larger change in demand than those with high time prices in response to a change in insurance.

Who are those with low time prices? One group consists of those with low values of w, that is, the poor. Another consists of those covered by sick-leave plans who do not lose wages from medical utilization. (For an individual who loses no wages from a physician visit, the effective value of w is zero.) Thus, our theory would predict that the poor might be quite responsive to changes in insurance, whereas the self-employed business-person or professional—who has a high value of w—might be little affected. Indeed, their demand could decrease if a general change in insurance causes t to rise.

The theory developed so far assumes a constant unit price for medical care P_M. Insight into real phenomena as well as practice in manipulating indifference curves can be gained by considering the effects of a health insurance policy with a deductible. Such a policy is moderately common. It says that the insurer will pay a certain percentage of all costs above $X per period (for example, 80 percent of costs above $100 per year), but that the individual must pay for the first $X. In this case medical care costs P_M per unit until $X has been spent on medical care; thereafter, it costs cP_M. How does this pricing structure modify our theory of demand?

Let us suppose that the deductible is a daily (and not an annual deductible. Then the effect of the deductible on quantity demanded is shown in Fig. 2.4. (Incidentally, Fig. 2.4 shows how any quantity discount, such as was formerly common in electricity pricing, would be diagrammed.) Between C and A, the consumer pays the full unit price; between A and M, the per-unit price is subsidized according to the terms of the insurance policy. In the illustration it is assumed that additional medical services cost 20 percent of the unit price (i.e., $c = 0.2$).

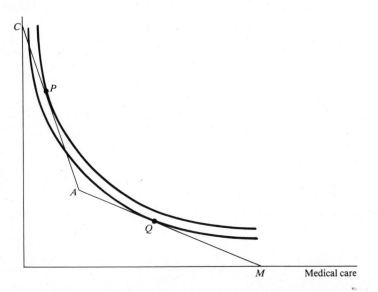

Fig. 2.4 With a deductible there are two local maxima. The line segment AC corresponds to expenditure before the deductible is reached, whereas the line segment AM corresponds to the budget constraint after the deductible is reached.

It is immediately apparent that there are two tangencies with indifference curves in this figure (points P and Q), although one of the tangencies represents a higher level of well-being than the other.[5] The maximum at P

5 In the language of the calculus, there are two local maxima and (in general) one global maximum.

represents a higher level of well-being than the one at Q, which means the consumer will choose not to exceed the deductible; however, the indifference curves could be drawn differently so that the consumer would choose to exceed the deductible. (Can you draw such indifference curves?) We can see that consumers will typically not be found purchasing near the "kink" (point A) in the budget line; in terms of the fuel example, if both electricity and natural gas sell for progressively declining unit prices, consumers will tend to specialize in one fuel and either principally use gas or principally use electricity in their homes.

A deductible in a health insurance policy is more complicated than the case just described, because the deductible typically applies not to a one-day period, but rather to several months at a time (frequently a year). Thus, if the bill for the doctor's visit made on the first day of the deductible period does not exceed the deductible, the expenditure will still apply toward the deductible, and future expenses (within the period) may be sufficiently large to exceed the deductible. In this case, how would a deductible affect demand?

A utility-maximizing consumer would act as if the following thought process were being pursued: If I knew with certainty that I would not exceed the deductible during this deductible period, the "true" price of this visit would be what I was charged. If, on the other hand, I knew with certainty that I would exceed the deductible, the "true" price of the visit would be only 20 percent of the stated price (if $c = 0.2$). Why? Suppose the doctor charges $10 for the visit. If I do not go to the doctor, I will have a certain amount of money at the end of the year. If I go to the doctor, that amount will not be $10 smaller, but will be $2 smaller because I will exceed the deductible anyway, and each extra visit ("the marginal visit") only costs $2. At the moment, it is uncertain whether or not I will exceed the deductible. The more likely I am to exceed the deductible, the closer is the true price of a visit to $2 and vice versa.[6] I am more likely to exceed the deductible if it is smaller (if I am closer to it) because the probability of being sick a few times is higher than the probability of being sick many times (alternatively, the probability of a minor or a serious illness is higher than that of only a serious illness). Also, I am more likely to exceed the deductible the more time is left in the deductible period (because I am more likely to be sick, the greater the length of time involved). Thus, the true price is lower the smaller the deductible, and the longer the period for which the deductible applies.

What are the implications of this discussion of deductibles? If deductibles are very large, the consumer is likely to behave as an uninsured con-

---

6 More exactly, the expected price is $(1 - p)P_M + pcP_M$, where p is the probability of exceeding the deductible and c is the coinsurance rate after the deductible. The theory of a deductible's effect on demand is more fully developed in [5].

sumer; because the probability of exceeding the deductible is (by definition) small, the true price is close to the stated price P_M. If deductibles are very small (or applied over a very long time period), the consumer is likely to behave as an insured consumer (i.e., no deductible), because the true price would be close to the insured price after the deductible. (Can you specify in theoretical terms the difference in demand between a policy with no deductible and a policy with a deductible that an individual would exceed with certainty? Hint: Because the true price is the same in each case, there is no substitution effect.) Thus the demand curve for medical services as a function of a deductible with a coinsurance rate c following the deductible is hypothesized to look like the curves shown in Fig. 2.5. For very large deductibles, the size of the coinsurance rate following the deductible matters little for demand. Nor will small changes in the deductible significantly affect demand. For very small deductibles the size of the coinsurance rate is quite important, although again, small changes in the deductible matter little.

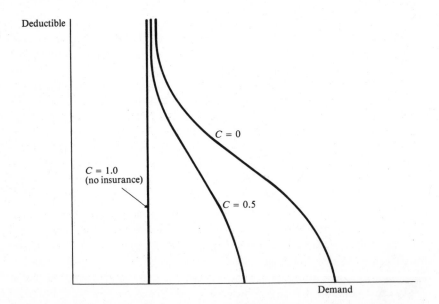

Fig. 2.5 The hypothesized shape of the demand curve with a deductible. The parameter c measures the fraction of cost left to the patient after deductible is satisfied.

What testable hypotheses has the theory of demand for medical care generated? First, the demand for care will respond to provisions of insurance coverage; specifically, the lower the coinsurance rate, the larger will be the demand. Second, other things equal, demand for care will be more responsive to changes in insurance among those with a low value of time.

Third, demand will not respond much to changes in a deductible for very small or very large values of a deductible, but (assuming near zero coinsurance above the deductible) there will be a range of deductibles within which demand may be quite responsive. In other words, the response of demand to variation in a deductible will be nonlinear.

EMPIRICAL EVIDENCE

More evidence has been generated concerning the first hypothesis, the responsiveness of overall demand, than either of the other two. There is enough evidence to regard the hypothesis that demand responds to changes in insurance as reasonably well established. Unfortunately, however, all the evidence regarding the first hypothesis is somewhat fragmentary and subject to criticism. A number of studies use methods similar to the Stanford study described above and compare behavior of groups who have different insurance plans. Two studies examined the demand for hospital services and found magnitudes of response to changes in coinsurance similar to those found in the Stanford study for physician services [6, 7]. Unlike the Stanford study, these studies of demand for hospital services suffer because the groups on the different insurance plans are different groups of people who have self-selected their insurance plan. We shall show later in this chapter that individuals who expect to be sick tend to purchase more extensive insurance, and therefore comparisons of different groups of individuals may be biased toward showing that insurance affects demand. Further, all the studies comparing groups on different insurance plans (including the Stanford study) are limited to specific ranges of coinsurance (in the Stanford example, from zero to 25 percent coinsurance), study specific medical services (for example, physician visits or hospital services), and study groups of individuals that are not necessarily representative of the entire population.

Another study used a quite different methodology to measure the responsiveness of demand to coinsurance. It analyzed insurance premiums for policies with coinsurance rates between 10 and 25 percent [8]. If demand did not respond to coinsurance, the ratio of the insurance company's payouts under the two plans should be 90/75. (With 10 percent coinsurance, the insurance company pays 90 percent, with 25 percent coinsurance it pays 75 percent.) If, however, demand varied with coinsurance, the payout under the 10-percent coinsurance plan would be more than 90/75 as large as the payout under the 25-percent coinsurance plan. (The insurance company would pay 90 percent of a larger total.) Premiums were obtained from four large insurance companies for policies with various coinsurance rates, and the implied responsiveness of demand (insurance elasticity of demand) was estimated. The responsiveness was somewhat smaller than, but close to, the elasticity generated from studies of groups on specific types of insurance plans.

Three criticisms may be made of this methodology. First, it relies on the assumption that the insurance company's loading charge (difference between premium and payout to insureds) was a constant fraction of the payout in policies with different coinsurance rates. Although there is some evidence to support this assumption (and it seems unlikely that the percentage would vary much over the range observed), there is no direct confirmation. More important, the calculations assume that the premiums were in fact based on the experience of the insurance company, as opposed to an actuary's "educated guess" of the responsiveness of demand. Finally, although the data do provide evidence that demand responds to insurance changes, the data come from the relatively narrow range of 10- to 25-percent coinsurance. If insurance plans were introduced with coinsurance values outside this narrow range, these data are of limited usefulness in predicting how demand might change.

Finally, some studies use data from household surveys to estimate how demand responds to insurance [9, 10, 11]. These studies have the advantage of utilizing a representative sample of the population, and they also typically have data on the socioeconomic characteristics of their subjects, so that it is easier to study whether the effect of an insurance change differs among groups. The magnitude of the elasticities estimated in these studies is roughly consistent with that estimated in other studies, although in this case there are even more severe analytical problems. Again, there is the possibility that the results are biased because individuals who expect to use more medical care choose more generous insurance plans. (When one uses statistical methods designed to adjust for such bias, the estimated responsiveness of demand is quite imprecise.) The price variable is also difficult to define. Unlike the other studies that typically compare a small number of plans differing only along a few dimensions (for example, the coinsurance rate), studies using a representative sample of the population must deal with all insurance plans in the community. Those plans typically differ along many dimensions. (For example, one plan may provide $300 for laboratory services per hospital stay, another may cover all laboratory services above $300 per year, a third may treat laboratory services as any other service that is subject to a deductible and coinsurance rate.) In this case it becomes quite difficult to describe the price of the medical service simply, yet such a description is necessary to the estimation process. In order to derive simple measures of price, one must make approximations that could well distort these estimates.

Despite the weaknesses of the varying approaches, a variety of studies using different methodologies come to similar conclusions concerning the responsiveness of demand to insurance. Such agreement among studies makes the first hypothesis reasonably well established; demand for a number of different medical services does respond to variation in the extent of

insurance coverage. (See [12] for a summary of this literature.) These findings reject the naive view that only sickness matters and that the physician
does not take account of the patient's insurance coverage in making decisions. In short, these data are consistent with the theoretical framework described above.

The second hypothesis is that changes in insurance coverage should
have a larger effect on those with low values of time than on those with high
values. There are substantially fewer data regarding this hypothesis. In the
Stanford study referred to earlier, female dependents were the only group
whose responsiveness to insurance (elasticity of demand) was notably different from the average; their elasticities were much larger. Our theory
would have predicted such a result if female dependents in this sample
tended to have lower prices of time than other groups. Unfortunately, we
do not know enough about the characteristics of this sample to determine if
female dependents' price of time was in fact lower.[7] We do know, however,
that certain fixed costs of employment must be paid if any work is done (for
example, the costs of travel to and from the place of work). Such costs do
not vary with the number of hours worked. Now consider a person choosing
whether to remain at home or enter the labor force. If the value of the person's time is higher in the labor force than at home, the person will consider
entering the labor force; however, the value of time (wage rate) must be sufficiently higher to recoup any fixed costs incurred when entering the labor
force that would not be incurred if the person remained at home. If other
factors are equal, those in the labor force will then show a higher value of
time than those not in the labor force, because their value will include the
recovery of fixed costs. Such a conclusion is consistent with the Stanford
study's finding of greater demand responsiveness among dependents.

Another study from Canada examined the effect of imposing a $1.50
charge for office visits and a $2 charge for hospital visits when services had
previously been free. The effect was larger on the poor than the nonpoor,
just as the theory would predict. Utilization of services among the poor declined 18 percent, as contrasted with a 6- to 7-percent decline for the nonpoor [13]. A study using American survey data [9] found very small changes
in the insurance elasticity of demand for physician visits as income changed;
the poor were slightly more responsive than the nonpoor. The amount of
evidence on the second hypothesis is thus small and clearly subject to criticism, but it does provide some weak support for the hypothesis.

The third hypothesis is that demand should be a nonlinear function of
levels of a deductible. Here there is only one study [14]. It supports the third

---

7 In particular, we do not know the education of the individuals in the sample or the
wages of others in the household.

hypothesis, although the amount of information available to construct estimates is scanty, and the findings must be regarded as very tentative.

A question one might raise is why this review of evidence has taken so
little account of foreign countries' experience. After all, many countries
have changed their insurance arrangements over time. Could not one study
the effects of such changes? The individual who is knowledgeable about
data will say that most changes occurred many years ago and results cannot
be confidently applied to today's world. (Additionally, in many cases data
from the period before the change simply do not exist.) The economist
would add that the observed changes in those countries reflect the interac-
tion of demand with a less than perfectly elastic supply curve. Consequently, the results do not reflect only the change in demand. The studies
summarized above, however, come from studies of groups in which the
change in demand changed the total demand in the market only negligibly,
so that the observed change in the behavior of the group can reasonably be
taken as measuring the change in demand.[8]

Data from Canada can, however, show how the medical care system re-
acts to a sudden increase in demand. When full coverage for ambulatory
services was introduced in Quebec, demand apparently exceeded the immediately available supply. As a result, the waiting time for an appointment in
Montreal nearly doubled (from six days to eleven days), the time physicians
spent per visit fell from nineteen to sixteen minutes, and the time patients
spent waiting in the office rose from thirty-six to forty minutes [15, 16].
That waiting time for an appointment increased so much more than waiting
time in the office suggests physicians kept their appointment system in
effect, but it became much harder to obtain an appointment.

In light of the fragmentary evidence concerning the demand for medical
services and the importance of the issue to public policy, the United States
Department of Health, Education, and Welfare is financing a social experiment to measure the responsiveness of demand to insurance, and to test
whether that responsiveness differs among income classes or other subgroups of the population [17]. As part of this experiment, around 7,000 persons in several areas of the country have agreed to change their insurance
for a period of three to five years. Some of these persons receive free medical care; others have a plan that approximates a large deductible; still others
have plans with coinsurance rates or deductibles intermediate between these
two extremes. The experiment acts as the participants' insurance company

8 The Canadian study cited above in support of the second hypothesis is an exception in that the utilization charges were imposed on an entire province, Saskatche-
wan. However, my use of the data was to show that the poor were differentially affected by the change in insurance rather than to quantify the extent of the change in
demand; for this purpose it is legitimate to use data from a case in which everyone's
insurance changed.

and in the process collects data on utilization. As a result, much more will be known about the demand for medical services and how it varies across different groups in a few years.

THE DEMAND FOR INSURANCE

Up to now we have assumed that the individual makes decisions about how much medical care to consume conditional upon owning a certain health insurance policy. Now we turn to the question of the selection of the insurance policy. First we take up the issue of how an individual might select a policy, and then we turn to the more complicated, but more common, case of group insurance.

The purpose of any insurance policy is to convert an uncertain, but potentially large, loss into a certain, small loss. Such a conversion benefits the consumer if greater losses cause progressively larger declines in utility (that is, if there is diminishing marginal utility to wealth). In this case the consumer's utility function will look like that shown in Fig. 2.6. Starting from the current position of wealth, OW, a loss is shown by a move from W toward the origin. Small losses (moves in the vicinity of W) cause relatively little loss in utility, but large losses of wealth cause disproportionately large losses in utility. Suppose the consumer is faced with the possibility of a loss that would move his or her wealth position to OX. Suppose the possibility of such a loss is 50 percent; without insurance, the consumer will have the utility level OM 50 percent of the time and utility level ON 50 percent of the

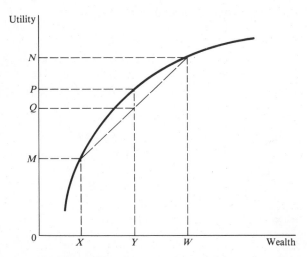

Fig. 2.6 The rationale for buying insurance. By paying a premium equal to WY, the consumer guarantees utility level OP, whereas without insurance, expected utility is OQ.

time. The consumer's average or expected utility is the average of *OM* and *ON*. This average is *OQ*. If, however, the consumer could buy insurance, it would cost an amount equal to *WY*, where *Y* is halfway between *W* and *X*, plus any fee the insurer charges for administrative costs and profits. Let us ignore the insurer's fee for the moment. After purchasing insurance the individual has wealth *OY* and utility *OP*. Because *OP* exceeds *OQ*, on a probabilistic basis the consumer is better off purchasing insurance. Such a conclusion depends only on the assumed shape of the utility function (diminishing marginal utility for wealth as wealth increases), and the assumption that the insurer's fee is sufficiently small so as to not wipe out the difference between *OP* and *OQ*. A consumer with the utility function diagrammed in Fig. 2.6 is said to be risk averse.

Figure 2.6 shows the rationale for any type of insurance. How does the reasoning apply in the case of health insurance? Recall that sickness was assumed to act like a random loss to the consumer; depending on how sick the person was, demand for medical care could be at various levels (Fig. 2.3). Moreover, because the consumer has fixed resources, consumption of other goods must be reduced, dollar for dollar, as medical expenditures rise. It seems reasonable to suppose that the consumer treats medical expenditures as occasioned by a random loss of health (just as repairs to a house might be desirable after a severe storm), and that to keep income available to spend on other goods and services relatively constant, the consumer insures against substantial decreases in wealth from illness.[9] Thus, if a woman requires breast surgery, her wealth position if she were not insured (after paying medical bills) might move to a point such as *OX* in Fig. 2.6. She therefore pays a small premium to protect against large losses.

Note that this theory can explain why a deductible might exist in a health insurance (or any kind of insurance) policy. To pay the insurance company a fee to insure the first few dollars of loss may not be worthwhile (the gap between the curved line and the straight line in Fig. 2.6 is not large in the immediate vicinity of *W*), although protection against a large loss may be much desired.

The theory emphasizes the importance of the insurance company's fee in determining demand. Empirical studies have verified its importance; the size of the loading fee is a critical determinant of the amount of health insurance demanded [18].

In practice, individual health insurance, which is relatively easy to analyze, is not widespread. Over 80 percent of the private health insurance in the United States is group insurance made available through the place of

---

9 Some argue that health insurance should be designed to promote health and not just a device to protect against losses in wealth. We consider the degree to which health services promote health in Chapter 5.

employment; that is, most people obtain health insurance as a fringe benefit from their employer. Health insurance is purchased through groups rather than individually for two reasons. First, employer-paid health insurance premiums are not taxable income to the employee. Hence, if the employee is going to purchase health insurance anyway, it is advantageous to take a portion of wages or salary in the form of employer-paid premiums; in effect, those dollars are before-tax dollars (because the premium is not considered part of wages by the Internal Revenue Service), whereas any premiums paid by the employee personally come from after-tax dollars (except that half of the premium may be deducted for households that itemize deductions).

A second reason for widespread group insurance is that adverse selection may eliminate the market for some kinds of individually purchased insurance. Suppose individuals differ in their risk because some are healthier than others. Further, suppose one knows more about one's own risk than an insurance company knows. To take an extreme case, suppose there are a number of individuals, half of whom are expected to spend $100 on medical care in a year and half of whom are expected to spend $300. An insurance company cannot distinguish the individuals, but they know their own risk. If all the individuals purchase insurance, the premium is based on their average expenditure, $200. However, such insurance will appear very expensive to those individuals who only expect to spend $100, and they may well not purchase it. If they do not, the insurance company is left insuring those individuals whose expenditure is $300 (at a premium based on expenditures of $300, which will make the insurance even less attractive to the better risks). The better risks will then not be insured.[10] If we generalize to situations in which individuals differ in their risks and no two individuals are alike (i.e., a "continuous" case), individual insurance may cease to exist altogether.

Adverse selection appears to be a real phenomenon. Health status partially determines the amount of insurance an individual has; the lower the self-rating of health status, the more insurance the individual is likely to own, other things being equal [18]. Some have attempted to explain as adverse selection the aged's difficulty in obtaining insurance prior to the Medicare program [19].

The problem of adverse selection is considerably eased if the insurance company insures an entire group that has been formed for reasons unrelated to insurance; for example, the employees of a company. Partly for reasons

---

10 In this situation a competitive equilibrium may not exist [19, 20]. An equilibrium would exist if no insurance policy exists whose expected profit is negative and no policy can be devised whose expected profit is nonnegative, given the policies that exist.

of adverse selection, group insurance requires that a certain percentage of the work force join the insurance plan (typically 75 percent). Because virtually all work-group insurance has some or all of the premium paid by the employer, obtaining high rates of participation is common.

We are left with the problem of explaining how much insurance is bought when the purchase occurs through the place of employment, and each employee is given the same insurance plan. Two explanations have been advanced [21]. The first emphasizes the employer's role in dividing compensation between cash and fringe benefits. Given the same total compensation by the employer, if a different mix between cash and fringe benefits would be desired by some employees, then it would pay another employer to offer the different mix (the second employer could obtain labor more cheaply). In equilibrium, each employer should be offering that mix of fringe benefits and cash desired by the employees. This view emphasizes the role of the *marginal employee* (the one who might change firms) in determining the terms of the group's health insurance policy.

The second view emphasizes the labor union's role. The union formulates a position on the division of compensation between cash payments and fringe benefits. If the union operates under democratic rule in formulating its position, it will follow the preferences of the *median member*. Otherwise a majority could be found to vote down the proposal.[11]

These two models of choice have different implications for the amount of group insurance purchased. In part because health insurance is probably more important to the median than the marginal employee, unions typically take more of their pay in the form of health insurance plans. Moreover, the amount of health insurance purchased in unionized firms rises much more with average wages than the amount purchased in nonunionized firms. This finding is consistent with the two models because the median wage is probably very close to the average wage, while the relationship between the average wage and the wage paid the marginal worker is probably much less.

To sum up this section, demand for health insurance can be viewed as attempting to convert a large potential random loss (caused by becoming seriously ill) into a small certain loss. Purchasing some insurance will improve the well-being (level of utility) of risk-averse consumers. How much insurance will be purchased depends importantly on the price of the insurance (the insurer's fee) and how risk averse the consumer is. A threat to an insurance market's existence arises if the insureds know more about their true risks than their insurance company. This is one rationale for providing either public insurance or private group insurance, as is the case for most

_____

11 Logrolling or agreements among members to vote in certain ways (vote-trading) may modify the outcome.

health insurance in the United States. Theories have been developed to explain how groups choose the amount of health insurance; these theories build on the theory of how an individual chooses insurance.

REFERENCES

1. Roger I. Lee and Lewis W. Jones. *The Fundamentals of Good Medical Care: An Outline of the Fundamentals of Good Medical Care and an Estimate of the Service Required to Supply the Medical Needs of the United States.* Chicago, Ill.: University of Chicago Press, 1933.

2. Hyman K. Schonfeld, Jean F. Heston, and Isidore S. Falk. "Number of Physicians Required for Primary Medical Care." *New England Journal of Medicine* 286, No. 11: 571-576 (16 March, 1972).

3. Ronald Andersen and Lee Benham. "Factors Affecting the Relationship between Family Income and Medical Care Consumption." In *Empirical Studies in Health Economics*, edited by Herbert E. Klarman. Baltimore, Md.: The Johns Hopkins Press, 1970.

4. Anne A. Scitovsky and Nelda M. Snyder. "Effect of Coinsurance on Use of Physician Services." *Social Security Bulletin* 35: 3-19 (June 1972).

5. Emmett B. Keeler, Joseph P. Newhouse, and Charles E. Phelps, "Deductibles and the Demand for Medical Care Services: A Theory of a Consumer Facing a Variable Price Schedule Under Uncertainty," *Econometrica* 45, No. 3: 641-655 (April 1977).

6. Charles T. Heaney and Donald C. Riedel. "From Indemnity to Full Coverage: Changes in Hospital Utilization." *Blue Cross Association Research Series 5.* Chicago, Ill.: Blue Cross Association (October 1970).

7. R. Williams. "A Comparison of Hospital Utilization by Costs and by Types of Coverage." *Inquiry* 3: 28-42 (September 1966).

8. Charles E. Phelps and Joseph P. Newhouse. "Coinsurance, the Price of Time, and the Demand for Medical Services." *Review of Economics and Statistics* 56, No. 3: 334-342 (August 1974).

9. Joseph P. Newhouse and Charles E. Phelps. "Price and Income Elasticities for Medical Care Services." In *The Economics of Health and Medical Care: Proceedings of a Conference Held by the International Economics Association at Tokyo*, edited by Mark Perlman. London: Macmillan, 1974.

10. Joseph P. Newhouse and Charles E. Phelps. "New Estimates of Price and Income Elasticities." In *The Role of Health Insurance in the Health Services Sector,* edited by Richard N. Rosett. New York: National Bureau of Economic Research, 1976. (Univeristies-National Bureau Conference Series No. 27.)

11. Charles E. Phelps. "Effects of Insurance on Demand for Medical Care." In *Equity in Health Services*, edited by Ronald Andersen et al. Cambridge, Mass.: Ballinger, 1975.

12. Joseph P. Newhouse, Charles E. Phelps, and William B. Schwartz. "Policy Options and the Impact of National Health Insurance." *New England Journal of Medicine* 290, No. 24: 1345–1359 (13 June, 1974).

13. R. G. Beck. "The Effects of Co-Payment on the Poor." *Journal of Human Resources* 9, No. 1: 129–142 (Winter 1974).

14. Joseph P. Newhouse, John E. Rolph, Bryant M. Mori, and Maureen Murphy. "An Estimate of the Impact of Deductibles on the Demand for Medical Care Services," forthcoming as R-1661-HEW, The Rand Corporation, Santa Monica, California.

15. Philip E. Enterline et al. "Effects of 'Free' Medical Care on Medical Practice—The Quebec Experience." *New England Journal of Medicine* 288, No. 22: 1152–1155 (May 31, 1973).

16. Philip E. Enterline et al. "The Distribution of Medical Services Before and After 'Free' Medical Care—The Quebec Experience." *New England Journal of Medicine* 289, No. 22: 1174–1178 (29 November, 1973).

17. Joseph P. Newhouse. "A Design for a Health Insurance Experiment." *Inquiry* 11, No. 1: 5–27 (March 1974).

18. Charles E. Phelps. "Demand for Health Insurance: A Theoretical and Empirical Investigation." The Rand Corporation, Santa Monica, California, R-1054-OEO, July 1973.

19. George A. Akerlof. "The Market for Lemons: Qualitative Uncertainty and the Market Mechanism." *Quarterly Journal of Economics* 84, No. 3: 488–500 (August 1970).

20. Michael Rothschild and Joseph Stiglitz. "Equilibrium in Competitive Insurance Markets: An Essay on the Economics of Imperfect Information." *Quarterly Journal of Economics* 90, No. 4: 629–650 (November 1976).

21. Gerald Goldstein and Mark Pauly. "Group Health Insurance as a Local Public Good." In *The Role of Health Insurance in the Health Services Sector*, edited by Richard N. Rosett. New York: National Bureau of Economic Research, 1976. (Universities-National Bureau Conference Series No. 27.)

Physician Supply   3

Within the confines of this book the supply of medical care cannot be treated comprehensively. Therefore, we will limit the discussion of supply to two topics, the financing of medical schools and determining the appropriate number of physicians to educate. Both represent problems of public policy about which economic analysis has something to say. Medical school financing and capacity are related topics, because a societal decision to increase (or decrease) the number of physicians being trained has implications for medical school financing. We take up the issue of financing medical schools first, after a brief discussion of recent legislative history that is applicable to both topics.

THE FEDERAL GOVERNMENT AND MEDICAL SCHOOLS

Throughout the 1950s and 1960s a body of opinion held that a physician shortage existed. This chapter's conclusion will examine the basis for this view, but enough people were persuaded of its validity that the federal government took action. It began to provide medical schools with funds to increase class size. In 1963 Congress enacted the Health Professions Educational Assistance Act, which provided the first substantial federal support for undergraduate medical training (i.e., training that leads to the M.D. degree). The act authorized grants to medical schools for 50 percent or more of the cost of new construction, renovations, and alterations. Additionally, the act authorized funds for a student loan program that enabled medical students to obtain loans at below-market interest rates. In 1965 a provision for scholarships, as well as loans, was added. At this time federal grants in support of operating expenses were also added. Most significantly, the 1965 amendments marked the first appearance of a so-called capitation payment.

Under this provision a medical school that wished to increase enrollment could apply for a grant that would provide a certain sum per student. In the first year of the capitation program (1966), the amount received per student among those schools that applied was roughly $200; in the next three years, this amount rose to roughly $550. The intent was to encourage expansion of class size. In addition, the 1965 amendments provided for a special grant to assist schools whose accreditation status was threatened by insufficient funds. Such grants were first used in 1968 and became known as financial distress grants.

In 1968 the manpower legislation was renewed, but capitation payments were made conditional upon further enrollment increases. First-year enrollment had to be increased by 2.5 percent or five students, whichever was greater. In 1970, $10 million in grant funds were earmarked for a program to expand medical school places by some 10 percent. In 1971, the manpower legislation was again up for renewal, but by this time, 62 of the 108 medical schools were receiving financial distress grants. Federal outlays for training physicians had been rising rapidly, from $237 million in fiscal year 1969 to $338 million in fiscal year 1971 [1]. A question arose as to how the federal government could be giving more money to medical schools, and yet more schools be in financial distress.

Some argued that provision of grants for distress encouraged distress; in effect, the federal government was in the position of underwriting additional expenditures that schools might wish to make. Partially for this reason, the 1971 act restructured the manner whereby the federal government gave money to medical schools. Grants for operating expenses and financial distress grants were terminated and were replaced with a much higher level of capitation support, an average of nearly $3,000 per student per year for students in four-year schools. By making a lump-sum amount available to the schools, the government sought to ease their financial burden, while not giving the schools a blank check for the federal Treasury. However, there was a string attached. To qualify for these monies, a school had to increase enrollment by 10 percent if the school had fewer than 100 entering students; otherwise, the increase had to be 5 percent or 10 students, whichever was larger. There was also a "bonus" if enrollment were increased still further. Thus for nearly a decade the federal government steadily increased monies going to medical schools if the schools would train more physicians. And as Table 3.1 shows, the schools responded.

FINANCING MEDICAL SCHOOLS

Given the new, much larger capitation grant of 1971, a question arose as to its appropriate size. The Congress desired to make the capitation grant equal to the cost of educating a medical student, and mandated in the 1971 act a study "to determine the national average annual per student educa-

Table 3.1 Medical school first-year enrollments

Year	Enrollment
1960–1961	8,298
1961–1962	8,483
1962–1963	8,642
1963–1964	8,772
1964–1965	8,856
1965–1966	8,759
1966–1967	8,964
1967–1968	9,479
1968–1969	9,863
1969–1970	10,401
1970–1971	11,348
1971–1972	12,361
1972–1973	13,726
1973–1974	14,185
1974–1975	14,963

Source: Anne E. Crowley, "Medical Education in the United States, 1974–1975," *Journal of the American Medical Association* 231 1337 Table 8 (December 1975).

tional cost of schools of medicine..." [2]. In this section we shall explore how one might have responded to the Congressional request to provide an estimate of educational cost.

Note first that Congress did not ask for the *change* in medical school costs if enrollment were increased a certain amount; it asked for the average (or per-student) cost. Below we shall argue that the change in costs, which we call the change in the pure cost of education, is the figure to use when contemplating a decision about expanding medical schools. But we shall also show that providing information about pure costs does not completely solve the problem of how to finance medical schools. Moreover, we shall see that attempts by government agencies that finance education to pay "only" the costs of education and agencies that finance patient care to pay "only" the costs of patient care can be self-defeating.

Medical school financing is a difficult conceptual issue because medical schools do more than produce education and so incur costs for reasons unrelated to education. Medical schools also treat patients and perform biomedical research. Sources of revenue show the importance of products other than education. Table 3.2 shows the sources of revenue for a sample of thirteen medical schools. While revenues received for education represent the single largest component of the medical school budget, they account for less than half of the total; research and patient care are also quite important.

Table 3.2 Sources of revenue for thirteen medical schools in 1972–1973

Source of revenue	Percentage of total revenue
Education	39
Tuition and fees	4
Gifts and endowments	5
Teaching/training grants	9
State appropriation	17
Federal capitation	4
Patient care	19
Research	33
Other	8
TOTAL	100

Source: Institute of Medicine, *Report of a study: Costs of Education in the Health Professions: Parts I and II,* January 1974. Washington, D.C.: National Academy of Sciences, 1974.

From whom do medical schools receive revenues? Much of their support comes from different levels of government. The federal government supports most of the research that is done; it also supports patient care through the Medicare and Medicaid programs, and education through the training grants and capitation programs. State governments support education, especially in state schools, and also support patient care through their share of the Medicaid program. Finally, local governments may support a certain amount of patient care, although their role is considerably smaller than those of the federal or state governments.

Because each government agency wants to pay only for the product it feels it is buying, how the medical school prices each "product" is important. For example, those government agencies supporting education wish to pay for education but not patient care or research, and the Medicare and Medicaid programs wish to pay for patient care, but not for the costs of education. It is partially for this reason that the Congress, when it contemplated a capitation grant program, wanted to know the cost of education.[1]

---

1 It may seem irrelevant to separate the cost of education from the cost of research and patient care if the government will pay the bill anyway. But which level of government pays the bill has important consequences for who in society finally pays the bill. For example, federal revenues are generally more progressive in their incidence than state and local revenues. Also, the Medicare program is primarily financed through a payroll tax, which is approximately proportional with respect to income, whereas research and education costs are financed out of general revenues, which are progressive with respect to income. Moreover, tuition, fees, gifts, endowment funds, and a considerable share of patient care revenues come from private sources, so that changing product prices can alter the share of total costs allocated to government.

From the point of view of economic theory, medical schools engage in joint poduction; that is, the same resource produces more than one product. A concrete example of joint production is a physician-in-chief conducting "rounds," that is, seeing various patients along with medical students (and house staff). The physician-in-chief is producing patient care (diagnosing and prescribing treatment for the patients seen) and also producing education (teaching the medical students by example). When joint production exists, one must take special precautions in specifying the cost of each product.

To illustrate the need for caution, we must define some terms. To make the discussion more concrete, we shall work through an example. Suppose a medical school produces only two products, teaching and patient care, and that its budget is $6 million. If the school's volume of patient care were produced without any education, assume that the total cost of patient care would be $3 million.[2] American medical education requires a certain minimum of patient care. Let us assume that if education were produced with this minimum amount of patient care, it would cost $5 million. These figures are shown in the first three rows of Table 3.3.

We now define the "pure" cost of Product A to be the additional or extra cost of producing Product A, assuming that all other products are at the minimum level possible, given the level of production of A. What is the

Table 3.3 Hypothetical example of joint production at a medical school

	Millions of dollars
Total cost of school	6
Cost if "school" produced only patient care	3
Cost if school produced only education	5
"Pure" cost of education*	3
"Pure" cost of patient care*	1
Joint costs *	2

*The pure cost of education is total cost (6) less the cost of producing only patient care (3). The pure cost of patient care is total cost (6) less the cost of producing only education (5). Joint costs are total costs (6) less all pure costs (3 + 1).

---

2 The $3 million figure is assumed to be the cost of producing equivalent quality patient care; if products whose costs are being compared are not similar, an adjustment must be made in the costs to make them similar.

pure cost of education for the school in Table 3.3? The present level of patient care would cost $3 million to produce if there were no education. But with the present level of education, the total cost of producing both is $6 million. Hence, education has added $3 million to total cost, and this value is the pure cost of education. We can similarly find a pure cost of patient care. If the present level of teaching were maintained with only the necessary minimum of patient care, cost would be $5 million. Treating additional patients adds $1 million to cost. These figures are shown in the fourth and fifth rows of Table 3.3.

Having worked our way through this semantic thicket, how can we use the concept of pure cost to illuminate the issue of interest to Congress—the cost of teaching medical students? The Congress could have specified (but did not) that it was interested in pure cost. For example, a study might have estimated the change of pure cost to increase enrollment by the amount Congress desired. This value would equal the costs of expanding medical schools, given that research and patient care remained at their present levels (or increased the minimal amount necessary to support the increased number of students). Instead, Congress asked for "the" cost of educating a medical student.

Existing studies of the cost of educating a medical student (including the study requested by Congress) have not used the concept of pure cost. Rather they employ an accounting approach that allocates all costs to a function (see for example [3]). For some costs allocation to one function is straightforward; for example, computer charges to perform research obviously are allocated to research. But other costs are not readily associated with one product (for example, a physician's conducting rounds); these costs are sometimes called overhead or indirect costs. Overhead costs arise in almost all firms, not just medical schools, and accounting conventions are typically used to allocate these costs among specific products, for example, the salary of the president of a firm may be allocated among several different products according to the revenues generated by each product. While this approach has the aesthetic appeal that all costs are allocated to one product or another, the resulting figures for "the" cost of any particular product are arbitrary; a different allocation convention would yield different costs for each product. In addition, an economist would argue that the resulting costs are not useful for making decisions about levels of production.

Two types of decisions must be made. One is expansion (or contraction) of a particular product. For this decision, changes in pure cost are relevant. Just as the firm examines marginal cost (and marginal revenue) in deciding whether to produce one more or one less unit, a firm producing joint products ought to weigh marginal revenue and changes in pure cost in examining the expansion of any single product. The second question is whether the entire enterprise should sink or swim; in this case, total cost is relevant. Even if it is worthwhile to expand the production of one kind of product because marginal revenue exceeds changes in pure cost, the firm should not be in business at all if total revenue falls short of total cost.

Because they use an accounting approach, existing studies of the cost of medical education ignore joint production and assign all costs to particular products through brute force. Frequently the researcher conducting the study circulates a questionnaire among faculty members, asking how they allocate time among teaching, research, and patient care. The faculty member might, for example, allocate one-third of total time to each. Although it is logically impossible in the case of joint production to arrive at a nonarbitrary allocation of time, the studies use the faculty members' responses to allocate faculty salaries among education, research, and patient care, just as if there were no joint production. As a result, studies that use this method will produce an arbitrary figure for the cost of education. Thus, when the Congress sets the size of the capitation grant on the basis of such studies, the grant amount is arbitrary. Should this be disturbing?

To answer that question, we need to consider the Congress's objectives. If it only wanted to induce schools to expand by paying the additional cost, it should have asked for the change in the pure cost of education that expansion would cause. Such an amount would by definition have covered the cost of the additional students.

Does it follow that Congress should be unwilling to pay more than pure cost for education, research, or patient care? The answer is no—to do so would carry a good thing too far. One can see in the example and show in a general case that the sum of pure costs will be less than the total cost.[3] In the example the sum of pure costs is $4 million and the total cost is $6 million. Thus, if this hypothetical medical school were reimbursed only for its pure costs, it would have a deficit of $2 million (called joint cost in Table 3.3). Such a deficit will always exist if it is advantageous to manufacture products jointly rather than separately. As a result, if all medical school "customers" (including government agencies) simply reimbursed the school for only the pure costs incurred by the activity that customer purchases, the medical

---

3 Let $TC(e, p)$ be a function that shows total costs as a function of the level of education and patient care. Let present production of education and patient care be at levels E and P, respectively. For the activities to be produced jointly, rather than separately, $TC(E, P) < TC(E, \bar{P}) + TC(O, P)$, where $\bar{P}$ is the minimal amount of patient care necessary to produce education. If we add the quantity $TC(E, P) - TC(O, P) - TC(E, \bar{P})$ to both sides of the inequality and rearrange, we have $(TC(E, P) - TC(O, P)) + (TC(E, P) - TC(E, \bar{P})) < TC(E, P)$. The two terms in parentheses on the left-hand side are the pure costs of education and patient care, respectively, so that the sum of pure costs is less than total costs. With more than two activities, it is necessary that all activities cost less jointly than separately. For a more detailed discussion, see [4].

school would be unable to pay its bills. But producing the activities together is cheaper than producing them separately, and so all parties willing to pay at least the pure cost must hope that someone will be willing to pay the joint costs.

In fact, that medical schools exist means someone pays the joint costs. A bargaining process among different government agencies probably determines who pays the joint costs. But the bargaining is not overt, and we know neither which agencies pay nor what part of joint costs private parties pay.

Thus we have reached the following conclusions. Given that the Congress was interested in expanding the number of places in medical schools, it should have asked for an estimate of change in pure cost. The decision to expand one product, however, differs from the decision to keep open the medical school's doors, and correspondingly different decision criteria must be used. If the criterion relevant to expanding one product (change in pure cost) were applied to reimbursement of all products (reimburse only pure cost), the medical school could not stay afloat. If no party is willing to pay more than the pure cost of a medical school's products, and other sources of support cannot be found (e.g., tuition, gifts), the school should probably not be in existence.[4]

Our analysis provides a different explanaton of why so many schools were in financial distress around 1970 (in addition to the argument that schools maximized revenues by claiming to be in distress). At that time there was a cutback in support for biomedical research; the extent of the decline in research revenues is shown in Table 3.4. To argue that this decrease caused the financial distress would be speculative. However, if the research funds were supporting a substantial share of joint costs, while education and patient care revenues more closely approximated pure costs, a cutback in research funds would indeed jeopardize the financial health of the medical school. Squeezing the research budget may have been like squeezing a balloon; if the balloon is not to break, the compression in one part of the balloon will appear as a bulge in another part, and the compression in the research sector may well have caused the education sector to bulge.

THE CAPACITY OF MEDICAL SCHOOLS

How many physicians should be trained? This question has provoked controversy for many years and merits a careful answer. The lengthy time necessary to train physicians makes it impossible to adjust to a shortfall

---

4 The "probably" appears in this sentence to take care of some assumptions that must be made to make a definite statement, but are beyond the scope of this chapter. They are touched on in a different context in Chapter 6.

Table 3.4 National institutes of health research obligations [1965 dollars]

Year	Millions of dollars	Percentage change from previous year
1965	831.5	
1966	894.7	+8
1967	951.3	+6
1968	952.3	0
1969	894.3	−6
1970	813.4	−9
1971	883.0	+9
1972	1046.1	+18
1973	1014.0	−3
1974	1244.5	+23
1975	1189.0	−4

Source: National Institutes of Health, "Basic Data Relating to the National Institutes of Health, 1976," Table 9.

quickly;[5] on the other hand, excessive numbers trained imply an excessive investment. Some would also argue that extra physicians create their own demand, a subject taken up in the next chapter. In addition to the issue of how many physicians to train, recent debate has centered on the distribution of physicians across specialties and geographic areas. Although I shall not discuss these two issues, one can use the analytical framework developed in this chapter to address them.[6]

The gestation period for a physician is indeed long. After four years of medical school and one more year of (graduate) training, a physician will

5 For the past several years a substantial part of new physician manpower consisted of foreign medical graduates (FMGs). For example, from 1965 to 1974, immigrant physicians were almost 42 percent of U.S. medical graduates [5, Table 2]. FMGs can be used to adjust for a shortfall quickly; thus the statement in the text needs to be qualified to say that it is impossible to adjust quickly with domestic graduates. The intent of recent legislation (P.L. 94–484) is to prevent FMGs from entering the United States permanently. Insofar as this objective is achieved, the qualification to the statement in the text is unimportant.

6 The analytic apparatus developed below applies directly to the question of geographic distribution; instead of considering the entire country as one market, the framework must be applied within each local market. The apparatus needs some generalization when applied to the specialty distribution issue. In particular, prices in all physician markets should enter the demand and supply functions. In technical terms, the partial equilibrium analysis presented below should be given a general equilibrium flavor by considering interrelationships among specialties. The reader who is interested in pursuing the subject of medical manpower further is referred to [6] and [7].

normally receive a license to practice medicine. Most physicians, however, take additional years of training. Including time required to construct training facilities and admit students, the time from a decision to increase the number of medical students to the time when those medical students are practicing medicine could well exceed a decade. Thus, the short-run supply of physicians at any point in time is nearly perfectly inelastic (what does the supply curve look like?); it has been effectively determined by the number of physicians that were trained a decade or more previously.[7] The question at hand is the number of physicians to train; that is, how many places there should be in medical schools.

In analyzing the issue of how many physicians to train, I shall assume that the appropriate number of medical students to train is that number that would be forthcoming if (1) students paid the pure cost (in the sense just described) of their education; and (2) at the time of making their occupational choices, students correctly anticipated the monetary and nonmonetary benefits that would accrue in the occupations considered. In short, I am making the assumption that the manpower planner should seek to train the number of physicians that would be forthcoming in long-run competitive equilibrium. Competitive equilibrium includes any effect of insurance on demand; thus, it is assumed that any demand induced by insurance should be satisfied. To be clear, I do *not* argue that the market for physician services is competitive; I only ask the manpower planner to train that number of physicians that would be trained in a competitive world.

Some would dispute the appropriateness of competitive analysis for this problem. Certain challenges to the applicability of competitive analysis are taken up in the next chapter, but I sketch here some of its desirable properties.

One such property is that any given level of physician services be produced at minimum cost. Even those who do not accept that a competitive equilibrium yields the right number of physicians would nevertheless agree that minimizing the cost of physician services (for each number of physicians trained) is desirable.

Another property creates more controversy. It is discussed more fully in Chapter 6, but the main idea can be profitably described here. In the previous chapter it was shown that the demand curve reflects the consumer's valuation of medical care relative to other goods and services. Given prices of medical care services and all other goods, the consumer chooses a mix of goods and services such that the last dollar spent on medical care buys as much utility as the last dollar spent on all other goods. Figure 3.1 shows a

---

7 This statement ignores variation in physician hours of work; however, physicians do not appear to vary their hours of work much in response to changes in hourly earnings; (8) and (9).

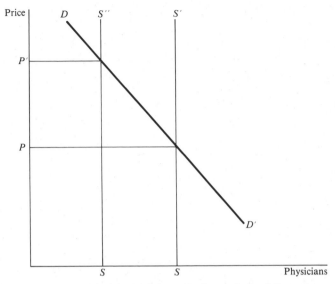

Fig. 3.1 Supply and demand for physicians. Both are derived from the supply and demand for physician services, which are assumed to be proportional to the number of physicians.

demand curve and two supply curves for physicians, the two supply curves corresponding to two different quantities of physicians being trained. Strictly speaking, demand is for physician services rather than physicians, but we shall suppose for the moment that each physician supplies a fixed number of services so that a given number of physicians always implies a certain number of physician-services, and vice versa. Suppose the number of physicians trained corresponds to the supply curve SS''. The equilibrium price is then P', and the last unit of physician services consumed will have a value to the consumer proportional to P'. If a larger number of physicians had been trained, equilibrium price would be P, and a larger number of services would be consumed, because some services are valued at an amount between P and P' (the nonzero elasticity and continuity of the demand curve guarantees this).

Consider now the prospective medical student who faces the cost of training and is interested in several aspects of possible occupations, including the monetary return. At higher prices (for example, P'), medicine will be a more attractive occupation, and more students will wish to enter it. Competitive equilibrium occurs when the price is maintained over time; that is, the number of entering students just offsets deaths, retirement, and any changes in demand and productivity.

Now we can see why a competitive equilibrium possesses desirable properties. Suppose the price is above the competitive equilibrium price; for example, suppose the capacity decisions at medical schools have been made such that the price is P', but that this price is above the long-run equilibrium price of P. Some students would have been willing to enter medicine given that the price was P' and are not admitted;[8] one can assume that some of these students would also have been willing to enter if the price were P. (That is, demand for medical education does not fall to zero if returns fall somewhat.) At the same time, there are consumers who would have been willing to pay an amount between P and P' for services. However, the shortfall in medical school places precludes an exchange between these consumers and the students who were not admitted. One can infer that the prospective physician and the prospective patient are both worse off, and no one else is made better off, because this exchange did not take place.[9] This is the desirable property of a competitive equilibrium.

Let us suppose then that the manpower planner has decided to emulate the competitive equilibrium solution in making a decision on the number of physicians to train. What problems must be solved in order to implement such a strategy? The planner must make a forecast of demand. If demand shifts, medical school capacity needs to change. How changes in price and income alter demand was discussed in the previous chapter; forecasting the effect on demand of changes in other variables, such as changes in age composition or health status, is conceptually straightforward, but cannot be described here because of space limitations. We shall, however, show below that correct estimates of demand would probably resolve the greatest uncertainty about how many physicians to train.

It may seem as though tracking demand ends the planner's task; if the number of physicians changes proportionately with demand, will that not preserve equilibrium? Unfortunately, the planner's problem is not nearly so simple.

To facilitate exposition to this point, we made an assumption that the number of physician services was proportional to the number of physicians. It is time to drop that assumption and look more deeply into the production of physician services. That look will reveal alternative methods for producing physician services that need consideration when the planner makes decisions on the number of physicians.

Let us suppose that a physician produces physician services by combining the physician's own time with nurses' time. (Nurses' time might include other support services, just as the composite commodity COMP in Chapter 2 included other goods.) Figure 3.2 illustrates two isoquants, the production equivalent of the indifference curves used in Chapter 2. The isoquants show

---

8 Remember that since P' is above the equilibrium price, in a competitive market additional supply would enter and the supply curve would shift out.

9 More precisely, no one else is sufficiently better off that they cannot be compensated. See Chapter 6 for a more rigorous argument.

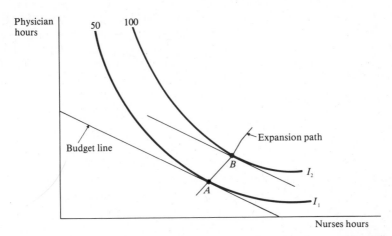

Fig. 3.2 Two isoquants, I_1 and I_2, for physician services showing combinations of physician hours and nurses hours that will produce 50 and 100 units of services respectively. The budget line is tangent to I_1 at point A. Why does the budget line slope sharply to the right?

substitution possibilities between nurse-hours and physician-hours in the production of physician services. Thus, with more physicians and fewer nurses, the same number of services could be produced; with more of both physician time and nurses time, more services could be produced.

What is the cost-minimizing mix of nurses and physicians? Just as in the analysis of the previous chapter, it is the point where the budget line is tangent to the isoquant (points A and B in Fig. 3.2). The budget line has a slope equal to (the negative of) the ratio of factor prices, that is, the ratio of the physician's hourly wage to the nurse's hourly wage. Is there an objection that physicians do not earn an hourly wage? For these purposes the physician "wage" in this ratio is the rate at which the physician would trade an hour not devoted to providing services ("leisure") to providing services. Further, it can be shown that a physician who maximizes utility will combine nurses' time and physician time in a way that minimizes the cost of producing a given bundle of services, that is, such a physician will produce at the point of tangency (see Chapter 4). The locus of tangencies as one shifts the budget line (two budget lines are shown in Fig. 3.2) is termed an expansion path. This path gives a relationship between total cost and quantity of production (from which comes the total cost curve). From the total cost curve can be derived a marginal cost curve (how?), and in a competitive industry the marginal cost curve is the supply curve (why?).

If such a supply curve can be estimated, we can broaden the planner's horizons to include more than forcasting demand. To derive the supply curve, the planner must know the location of the isoquants. Over time, as technology changes, the isoquants may shift in toward the origin, so that more services can be delivered from a given number of person-hours. Thus, the planner must know the rate of technological change in the production of physician services in order to judge the appropriate number of physicians to train. In practice, the rate of technological change is difficult to forecast, and most analysts assume that the isoquants will shift in each year at some constant rate (for example, 2 percent). Unfortunately, we do not have good measures of the magnitude of this shift, and even a small difference in the rate can have substantial consequences over a period of years. For example, a 3-percent rather than a 2-percent rate of shift, if maintained over ten years, means that 9 percent fewer physicians will be needed to produce the same mix of services. However difficult the task, a forecast of technological change must be made when making a decision on number of physicians to train.

The planner must know not only how fast technology will change, but also the specifics of the existing technology. Figure 3.2 alerts us to the possibility that there is more than one way to increase (or decrease) the production of physician services. Perhaps it would be less costly to increase physician services by increasing the number of nurses' hours available than by increasing the number of physician hours.

In fact, such a position has been taken by Uwe Reinhardt [10], who has estimated a production function for physician services. Figure 3.3 shows the actual isoquants for general practitioner office visits that Reinhardt estimated. These isoquants represent the technology available to produce physician visits in the mid-1960s. Aides include registered nurses, medical technicians, and clerical staff. Office hours per week represent physician hours. Output is measured as visits per week. Although Reinhardt does not draw the budget line, he argues in effect that it is not tangent to the isoquant at the starred points (which represent the current mix of aides and physicians on average) but has a flatter slope than the isoquant at that point. A hypothetical line of this type has been drawn. If Reinhardt's argument is correct, the same number of services could be produced with fewer physicians (and more aides), and the total cost of physician services would be lower. Can you find the cost-minimizing point?)

Now suppose the planner forecasts a demand increase and therefore wishes to supply more physician services. Reinhardt's argument implies that the cheapest way to expand physician services is not to add physicians, but to add aides. Why is this? The cheapest way to produce services is always at the point of tangency between the budget line and the isoquant. Therefore, the locus of tangencies (the expansion path) is the optimal mix of aides and physicians. (You can test your understanding by drawing in the expansion path.) According to Reinhardt's estimates, the current position lies to the left of the locus. Therefore, if more aides are added to a given number of physician hours, one will move toward the locus of tangencies. Only after one has reached it should further expansion of services use more physicians

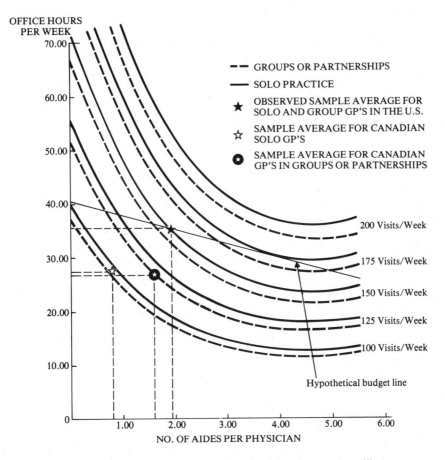

Fig. 3.3 Estimated feasible tradeoffs between physician time and auxiliary person-nel, general practitioners. (Reprinted with permission from *Physician Productivity and the Demand for Health Manpower* by Uwe E. Reinhardt. Copyright 1974, Bal-linger Publishing Company. The solid straight line has been added.)

(and still more aides). Reinhardt estimates that the optimal (cost-minimiz-ing) mix would roughly double the present number of aides per general practitioner and reduce the number of general practitioners by one-third. He reaches similar conclusions about pediatricians, obstetricians-gynecolo-gists, and internists. Thus, if correct, Reinhardt's estimates imply that the number of physicians already exceeds the number that would minimize the cost of the present level of (outpatient) physician services. But are his esti-mates correct?

Unfortunately, there is almost certainly a bias in Reinhardt's figures such that aides will be estimated to have a higher productivity than they in fact have. Reinhardt is aware of this problem, and argues that the extent of the bias is not quantitatively important. Because the point is critical, and because this example illustrates how biases can enter when estimating theoretical concepts from actual data, a look at Reinhardt's procedures is worthwhile.

In Fig. 3.4 the two curved lines illustrate two total revenue product curves for two different physicians. The vertical axis measures the physicians' revenues and costs, while the horizontal axis measures the number of aides. The slope of the total cost line equals the wage of an aide. (Why?) The physician is assumed to act as if the difference between total revenue and total cost is maximized. (Chapter 4 shows that a physician who maximizes utility would behave in this way.) The maximum difference occurs where the slope of the total revenue product curve equals the slope of the total cost line. (Why?) For Physician 1, this occurs at point A, so Physician 1 employs OE number of aides at a cost OC and makes a profit equal to AC. Suppose, however, that physicians vary in the effectiveness with which they can use aides, and that Physician 2 can manage aides better than Physician 1. Physician 2's total revenue produce curve is shown as lying above Physician 1's curve. To maximize profit, Physician 2 employs OF number of aides at a cost OD and makes a profit equal to BD.

Reinhardt estimates the productivity of physicians and aides by observing how many hours various physicians work, how many aides they use, and how many visits they produce. Thus, Reinhardt would observe Physician 1 at point A and Physician 2 at point B. He would then conclude that if a

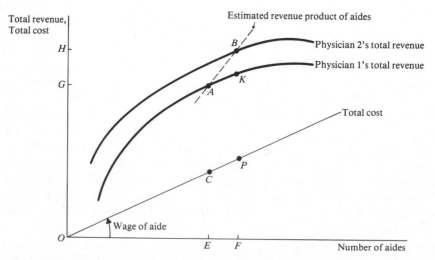

Fig. 3.4 Hypothetical total revenue product and total cost curves of aides for two hypothetical physicians showing how estimated productivity of aides may be biased upward. The dashed line through A and B shows the estimated revenue product curve.

physician were practicing with the number of aides equal to *OE*, an expansion to *OF* would raise total revenue (total visits) by the difference in revenues at points *A* and *B*, that is, *OH* minus *OG*. This, however, could drastically overstate the effectiveness of additional aides, for if Physician 1 and 2 actually added aides, they would in fact move along their respective total revenue product curves. For example, Physician 1 would move from point *A* to point *K*, so that the estimated marginal productivity of aides would be overstated by an amount equal to *BK*.

This type of bias occurs frequently in empirical analysis of production. We observe different firms in different positions. We wish to infer something about the technology (the production function) from observing the firms. However, if every firm faces the same technical possibilities (production function) and the same factor and product prices, all firms should be at the same point (or they would not be maximizing profits). That they are not at the same point indicates that something among them differs. If what differs is their ability to use factors productively, then there is a bias in inferring the technology. If, however, they face different factor or product prices, then there is no bias. In fact, this is the crux of Reinhardt's defense of his estimates; he argues that most of the differences among physicians are differences in product and factor prices rather than their ability to use aides.[10] If Reinhardt's argument is accepted (and one cannot generate any quantitative evidence to support or refute it), then it follows that the bias is small.

Suppose we accept Reinhardt's argument that the bias is small. Then his estimates imply that there are too many physicians producing the existing level of services. Does this mean that the decade-long expansion of medical schools should not have taken place? An answer requires some additional preparation.

Economists call the above analysis normative; it analyzes what should be (what is optimal). In this case it seeks to answer the questions: How many physicians should be trained? How many aides should be employed? Another branch of economics is positive analysis; it attempts to explain what actually is. In this case, it seeks to answer such questions as: How would employment of aides change if their wages changed? Positive analysis starts with the presumption that individuals maximize their utility (or that firms maximize profits) and uses such an assumption to derive testable predictions. Positive analysis would predict that physicians are at (or near) a cost-minimizing point. That prediction appears to be rejected by Reinhardt's estimates. In such a case one may reject the theory or question the estimates.

---

10 If physicians differ in their ability or willingness to maximize profits, the bias is further reduced.

We have already discussed one reason for questioning the estimates. As shown by Fig. 3.4, there may be a bias in the estimates, and the observed point may in fact be a cost-minimizing point.

Even assuming a negligible bias, however, the apparent failure to find cost minimization may be deceiving, for some costs may not have been counted. If there is a cost to the physician of managing more aides (it may take more time, or the physician may suffer psychic losses from delegating tasks), then the budget line that has been drawn is incorrect; accounting for any such costs could reveal that the current situation is consistent with the physician's maximizing utility. (How would the budget line in Fig. 3.3 look if these costs were accounted for?) Positive analysis thus alerts us to ask the questions: Why are phenomena the way they are? What is the mechanism that leads to an apparent nonoptimal outcome? If we cannot identify such a mechanism, we need to consider the possibility that our analysis is in error and the present situation is optimal. In that case, intervention with the intent of improving the outcome will only worsen it.[11]

Normative analysis thus must consider the possibility that the observed situation represents an optimum. The existence of management consulting firms, however, testifies that the situation prior to analysis does not always represent an optimum. In fact, economic theory predicts that events tend toward the optimum or the point of tangency, not that the optimum always obtains; only in a world where information and adjustment to changed circumstances are costless would one expect always to observe the tangency solution.

What then does a manpower planner make of Reinhardt's estimates? One possibility is that physicians simply do not know that adding aides will increase utility and that Reinhardt has played the role of management consultant. In this case dissemination of the information should increase the demand for aides, and over some range increases in demand for physician services could be met without new physicians. Too many physicians were trained given the present level of services. A second possibility is that dissemination of Reinhardt's results will not increase demand for aides because employing more aides will increase psychological or time costs. If time costs are increased the present situation may be optimal, and the present number of physicians is not necessarily excessive. If the costs are psychological, a more competitive market for physician services would probably increase the demand for aides. Physicians who were more willing to bear such costs could effectively undersell physicians who were less willing. Why this does not occur now is taken up in Chapter 4 and methods for making the market more competitive are taken up in Chapter 6. Thus if the market were made more competitive or if physicians were ignorant of

---

11 Although too conservative a decision rule, the traditional physician motto *Primum non nocere* ("Above all do not harm") conveys the same spirit.

the utility-maximizing employment of aides, the current level of services could probably be produced with fewer physicians.

STUDIES MADE BY PREVIOUS MANPOWER PLANNERS

We are now in a position to appraise the methodology used by studies that led to the expansion of medical schools during the 1960s. Examination of their methods is useful because such methods are often applied to all types of manpower planning, not just to medical manpower. These studies did not employ the competitive equilibrium solution as a criterion to emulate, and did not consider alternative techniques for producing physician services.

The first study of how many physicians should be trained was referred to in the previous chapter. In 1933, Roger Lee and Lewis Jones argued that approximately 135 physicians per 100,000 population were needed [11]. This figure was derived by soliciting experts' opinions of the number of hours needed to treat the health problems of a given population appropriately; the 135 per 100,000 figure indicated that the number of physicians trained should be somewhat increased.

A second important study was made by the President's Commission on the Health Needs of the Nation in 1953 [12]. This commission did not use the method of Lee and Jones, but rather examined existing physician/population ratios in various regions. The commission then projected the total number of physicians that would be required to maintain existing ratios nationwide given future population increases. It also projected the number of physicians needed to bring regions whose physician/population ratios were below the national average up to the national average. Both figures implied a need to train more physicians. A similar methodology was used by the Surgeon General's Consultant Group on Medical Education, who issued a report in 1959 [13]. This group began with the assumption that the demand (and need) for medical care would rise, and concluded that it would therefore be necessary at least to maintain the current ratio of physicians to population. To maintain the ratio required an increase in the number of physicians trained. It was against the background of these reports that the Kennedy Administration introduced legislation to expand medical schools, with the results described at the beginning of this chapter.

The drive to expand medical schools received further impetus from the *Report* of the National Advisory Commission on Health Manpower issued in 1967. This commission recommended ''a substantial expansion in the capacity of existing medical schools'' and ''continued development of new schools'' [14, p. 19], because it judged the delays in obtaining physician appointments as too lengthy. Following the commission's *Report*, Congress enacted the 1968 health manpower legislation that made capitation payments to medical schools conditional upon enrollment increases.

It is easy enough to see what may be wrong with the methods of these studies; indeed, some of the failings were noted at the time the policies to expand medical schools were adopted [15]. Before reading further, you might try to develop your own list of the difficulties that could arise in making decisions on medical school capacity using the methodologies just described. Some of the difficulties include the following:

1. The aim of training the number of physicians needed to treat a population ignores demand. So too does the aim of raising areas with fewer than average physicians to the national average. If additional physicians are trained because they are needed (as defined in [11] or [16]), there is no guarantee that anyone will enter the physician's office to be treated. Some would also argue that physicians might then create their own demand by recommending treatment in cases where treatment was of little or no value. Note that such makework could exist and professional judgment might still hold that some parts of the population were not receiving adequate care. Studies that do not account for demand inherently run the risk of wasting resources, because underutilized physicians represent resources that society could have used to accomplish other purposes.

2. Of those studies that do consider demand, most assume that demand for physician services changes only if the total population changes. Because demand for physician services varies markedly by age group, any shift in the age composition of the population will also lead to different demands on the medical care system. Additionally, demand may change within a given population because of changes in insurance coverage, as the last chapter pointed out.

3. Studies that use as a criterion existing ratios of physicians to population assume that the existing ratio is optimal. In fact, as Reinhardt argued, it may not be. Further, technological change may occur that would alter the desirable ratio. For example, development of a polio vaccine reduced the demand for physician services to treat polio.

4. Most of the studies cited assume that the supply of physician services is proportional to the number of physicians, but such an approximation may not be satisfactory. The supply of physician services is not proportional to physician hours (because of diminishing marginal productivity), and physician hours are not necessarily proportional to the number of physicians; if the proportion of part-time or retired physicians changes, the relationship between physician hours and the number of physicians will change.

5. Queues to see physicians do not by themselves establish that more physicians should be trained. Demand for physicians will fluctuate over time because of the random nature of illness. A system that minimizes the cost (including the cost of waiting time) of delivering any service for which demand fluctuates over time will occasionally have queueing because it is

cheaper to have some waiting than to staff for the peak load. Consider the examples of toll booths on the George Washington Bridge. Ensuring that a driver could always find an empty booth at rush hour would require an inordinate number of booths.

ARE WE TRAINING TOO MANY PHYSICIANS?

If the historical studies have used inappropriate methodology, what would the appropriate methodology have told us? The question cannot be answered without some assumption about the desired level of demand. How to judge the desired level of demand is taken up in Chapter 6. Let us suppose here that the present level of demand is desired. Then Reinhardt's estimates imply that the expansion of medical schools described in Table 3.1 was possibly inappropriate, especially if policies are instituted to make the market for physician services more competitive (see Chapter 6). But the monies that trained existing physicians are sunk costs. What does appropriate methodology tell us about the future? Should the expanded level of medical school places be maintained?

Recall that the manpower planner should consider demand, technological change, and substitution possibilites. The planner should also account for additional physicians from foreign medical schools, but we shall assume the policy decision to reduce the numbers of such physicians to a very small number is effective (see note 1 of this chapter), and so ignore this source of supply.

Table 3.5 displays Reinhardt's estimates of the number of office-based physicians required to meet two levels of demand in 1990. The numbers, of course, vary depending on the assumed employment of aides. It is difficult to project the supply of office-based physicians in 1990, but the figure is likely to be in the range of 373,000 to 409,000.[12] Reinhardt's estimates show that this many physicians would be required if demand grew roughly 3 percent per person per year (to be 80 percent greater than 1970 levels) and

---

12 These figures are based on the American Medical Association's estimate of the number of physicians who have finished graduate training [17, Table 1]. The authors present a low and high estimate of physicians projected to 1985; the low estimate assumes that class sizes remain at 1976–1977 levels, and the high estimate assumes class sizes increase at the rate anticipated by medical schools. The low estimate projects an increase of 10,000 physicians per year between 1981 and 1985, and the high estimate projects an increase of 15,000 physicians per year. I have simply extrapolated this absolute rate of increase from 1985 to 1990. One must then estimate the number of office-based physicians from the number of total physicians. To do this I have used figures from Katz, Warner, and Whittington [18, Tables 1 and 2] and calculated that 76 percent of total active physicians who were not in graduate training in 1976 were in office-based practice. I have then assumed that a similar portion will be in office-based practice in 1990.

Table 3.5 Office-based physicians required in 1990 depends on demand and use of aides [number of physicians in '000s]

Demand level in 1990	Aides per M.D.			
	Current level (1.75)	2.0	3.0	4.0
1970 level of per capita demand, 4.6 visits per person per year*	231	217	176	152
3% annual growth in per capita demand, 8.3 visits per person per year	421	396	321	276

Source: Uwe Reinhardt, *Physician Productivity and the Demand for Health Manpower.* Cambridge, Mass.: Ballinger, 1975.
*The 1975 level was 5.1 visits per person per year, roughly a 2-percent annual growth from 1970. See National Center for Health Statistics, "Current Estimates from the Health Interview Survey—United States" 1975; Washington, GPO, 1977 (DHEW Publication No. (HRA) 77–1543).

there were little or no substitution of aides for physicians. Several factors make this number of physicians seem too large.

1. An 80-percent increase in demand seems high. Because my interest is to illustrate methods, I have not made a careful estimate of the change in demand, but some comments are germane. The growth in demand will be sensitive to how much insurance the population has. Demand for ambulatory services could grow by 80 percent over 1970 levels if the entire population has complete insurance coverage [19], but complete insurance is an extreme case. Moreover, demand for inpatient physician services will exhibit a smaller response to complete insurance because these services are now more extensively insured. Increases in income and the number of aged will cause demand to increase, but rough calculations suggest that the increase caused by these two factors will be on the order of only 20 percent.[13] Visit rates grew by only 11 percent between 1970 and 1975, well below a rate of growth necessary to achieve an 80 percent demand increase by 1990.

2. Reinhardt's assumptions about technological change (different methods of production) seem conservative. He explicitly does not consider the introduction of physician extenders, physician assistants, or other types of allied health personnel who have more training (and hence can do more) than

13 An increase in real income of 3 percent per year and an income elasticity of 0.2 [20] will increase demand by around 16 percent. The visit rate among the aged is some one-third greater than among the nonaged [21]; an increase in their share of the population from 10 to 20 percent will increase demand only 3 percent.

traditional allied health personnel (primarily nurses). To the degree such personnel are introduced, fewer physicians are needed.

3. With 400,000 physicians, little or no increase in aides per physician will be necessary, yet markedly fewer physicians are required if aides can be substituted.

4. The assumptions about the number of foreign medical graduates are conservative. If foreign medical graduates continue to enter in spite of current intentions, there will be still more physicians than projected.

For all these reasons, there is a good case that we are training too many physicians. If so, it would be eloquent testimony to making public policy decisions using unsound methodology.

REFERENCES

1. Office of Management and Budget. *Special Analysis: Budget of the United States, Fiscal Year 1971.* Washington: Government Printing Office, 1970, p. 152.

2. Public Law 92-157, Section 205(a)(1).

3. Institute of Medicine. *Report of a Study: Costs of Education in the Health Professions: Parts I and II, January 1974.* Washington: National Academy of Sciences, 1974.

4. John E. Koehler and Robert L. Slighton. "Activity Analysis and Cost Analysis in Medical Schools." *Journal of Medical Education* 48, No. 6: 531–50 (June 1973).

5. Bureau of Health Resources Development. "Foreign Medical Graduates and Physician Manpower in the United States." Washington: Government Printing Office, 1974 (DHEW Publication No. (HRA) 74–30).

6. Judith R. Lave, Lester B. Lave, and Samuel Leinhardt. "Medical Manpower Models: Need, Demand, and Supply." *Inquiry* 12, No. 2: 97–125 (June 1975).

7. *Health Manpower and Productivity: The Literature and Required Future Research,* edited by John Rafferty. Lexington, Mass.: D. C. Heath, 1974.

8. Frank A. Sloan. "A Microanalysis of Physicians' Hours of Work Decisions." In *The Economics of Health and Medical Care: Proceedings of a Conference Held by the International Economics Association at Tokyo,* edited by Mark Perlman. London: Macmillan, 1974.

9. Stephen G. Vahovich. "Physicians' Supply Decisions by Specialty: 2SLS Model." *Industrial Relations* 16, No. 1: 51–60 (February 1977).

10. Uwe E. Reinhardt. *Physician Productivity and the Demand for Health Manpower.* Cambridge, Mass.: Ballinger, 1975.

11. Roger I. Lee and Lewis W. Jones. *The Fundamentals of Good Medical Care: An Outline of the Fundamentals of Good Medical Care and an Estimate of the Service Required to Supply the Medical Needs of the United States.* Chicago: University of Chicago Press, 1933.

12. President's Commission on the Health Needs of the Nation. *Building America's Health,* Vol. 2. Washington: Government Printing Office, 1953.

13. Surgeon General's Consultant Group on Medical Education. *Physicians for a Growing America.* Washington: Government Printing Office, 1959.

14. *Report of the National Advisory Commission on Health Manpower, Volume I.* Washington: Government Printing Office, 1967.

15. Rashi Fein. *The Doctor Shortage.* Washington: The Brookings Institution, 1967.

16. Hyman K. Schonfeld, Jean F. Heston, and Isidore S. Falk, "Numbers of Physicians Required for Primary Medical Care." *New England Journal of Medicine* 286, No. 11:571 (16 March, 1972).

17. American Medical Association. *Profile of Medical Practice, 1977.* Chicago: American Medical Association, 1977.

18. Martha Katz, David C. Warner, and Dale Whittington, "The Supply of Physicians and Physicians' Income: Some Projections." *Journal of Health Politics, Policy, and Law* 2, No. 2: 227–256 (Summer 1977).

19. Joseph P. Newhouse, Charles E. Phelps, and William B. Schwartz. "Policy Options and the Impact of National Health Insurance." *New England Journal of Medicine* 290, No. 24, 1345–1359 (13 June, 1974).

20. Ronald Andersen and Lee Benham. "Factors Affecting the Relationship between Family Income and Medical Care Consumption." In *Empirical Studies in Health Economics,* edited by Herbert Klarman. Baltimore: The Johns Hopkins Press, 1970.

21. National Center for Health Statistics. "Current Estimates from the Health Interview Survey: United States, 1975." Washington: Government Printing Office, 1977 (DHEW Publication No. (HRA) 77–1543).

The Medical   4
Marketplace

In this chapter we analyze the functioning of the medical marketplace. Some find it repugnant to think of medicine as a marketplace, perhaps because that conjures up images of haggling with a peddler over the price of some object, an image quite inconsistent with that of the healing hand. Nonetheless, medicine does resemble other markets in the economy. Most importantly, resources are used to produce medical services that could be used to produce other types of goods and services.

In the American economy, signals sent by market forces (especially prices) govern the amount of resources in medical care (and thereby determine what is available for other purposes). Such signals also govern the amount of medical care produced from a given set of resources, that is, the efficiency of production. The workings of market signals in medical care are the subject of this chapter. Thus, our study of the medical marketplace is also a study of the system of signals sent to physicians, patients, and other actors concerning decisions on the use of medical care resources.

Before discussing particular characteristics of the medical marketplace, it will be useful to review briefly the functions of an ideal market. In such a market consumers are assumed to come to the market with well-defined preferences. These preferences, together with prices and income, lead to a demand curve, showing how much consumers are willing to pay for various quantities of goods (see Chapter 2).

Consumers in an ideal market are assumed to be able to purchase goods and services from a variety of suppliers. Because consumers attempt to maximize utility given their income levels, they wish to find the lowest cost supplier of the desired good or service.

Suppliers of goods and services are assumed to maximize profit. As a result, suppliers have an incentive to produce the quality (or range of qualities) that consumers want to purchase; if a supplier does not do so, another supplier could take business away. Likewise, suppliers have an incentive to produce their goods and services at the minimum possible cost; otherwise, they can be undersold. If there is an inefficient group of suppliers in an industry, it is assumed that other firms from outside the industry will enter the market in pursuit of profits, thereby ensuring that those goods consumers most wish to purchase with their incomes are produced at a minimum cost.

The medical market place clearly differs from this idealized model. Some differences that have been frequently mentioned include:

1. Physicians and other suppliers are not interested solely in maximizing profit; they are also concerned with their workload.

2. Entry into medicine is restricted because one must have a license to practice. In order to obtain a license, one must either attend an American medical school, where the number of places are rationed, or undertake the additional expense and inconvenience of seeking a medical education abroad.

3. Consumers are ignorant about their medical needs; whereas they possess the knowledge to decide, say, whether they prefer an apple or a banana, they do not know whether they could profit from a particular therapeutic regimen. The usual presumption that the consumer knows best and so consumer demands should be satisfied (consumer sovereignty) is therefore not correct.

4. Partly because of consumer ignorance, suppliers can create their own demand. In particular, if providers are not fully occupied, they will attempt to create business for themselves by systematically misinforming the consumer. Consumer demands are thus not independent of suppliers, and for this reason also there is no presumption that those demands should be satisfied.

5. Because of the way in which medical insurance is structured, price competition has been severly undermined. The outcome of the medical marketplace therefore does not approximate that of a competitive market.

In the remainder of this chapter we shall discuss these objections. Most of our attention will be paid to the last two objections; we shall return to the third objection in the last chapter.

DO PHYSICIANS MAXIMIZE PROFITS?[1]

The standard theory of the firm assumes that firms maximize profits. Physicians, dentists, and other medical care providers form much of the

---

1 Differences between a nonprofit hospital and a for-profit firm are discussed in the Appendix to this chapter.

medical care industry. It is more reasonable to assume that they maximize their utility (taking account of their leisure) than to assume that they maximize profits. Suppose we relax the assumption of profit maximization and substitute maximization of utility. Would any results change?

Let us assume that physicians' utility functions include leisure and net income from their practices, and that they seek to maximize utility (subject to the demand curve they face and the constraint that there are but twenty-four hours in a day). Under these assumptions physicians will seek to minimize the cost of producing services (for a given number of hours of their own labor), because any monies saved will increase their net incomes. Hence, the predictions of a utility-maximizing model for employment of other factors of production (e.g., nurses) are the same as for a profit-maximizing model. Specifically, physicians will employ factors of production up to the point where their marginal revenue product (the amount of revenue produced from employing an addition unit) equals their marginal factor cost (the cost of employing an additional unit). If this were not the case, physicians could increase net income (and thereby utility) by altering the amount of factors employed.

The critical issue concerns the physicians's own hours of work.[2] Does the physician work fewer hours if we assume utility maximization than if we assume profit maximization? For simplicity we assume all time is spent in either work or leisure. Suppose the dependence between a physician's net professional income and hours of work is given by the curve ABCD in Fig. 4.1.[3] Point A on this line represents no hours devoted to practicing medicine (all time given to leisure) and no income from medicine. As hours practicing medicine increase (moving from right to left), net professional income also increases, though at a decreasing rate. From the utility function one can derive the physician's indifference curves between income and workload. The utility-maximizing physician will select hours of work (leisure) in order to reach the most northeastward indifference curve; this will occur when curve ABCD is tangent to an indifference curve, as at point B. The point of tangency clearly does not correspond in general to the net income-maximizing point, which on curve ABCD is represented by point C. (Net income falls after point C because it is assumed the physician cannot effectively work twenty-four hours per day.) Does this mean the utility-maximizing physician works less than the profit-maximizing physician?

Recall that the profit-maximizing firm maximizes the residual after the entrepreneur (physician) has paid himself or herself a wage sufficient to stay

---

2 The discussion that follows is based on [1].

3 Suppose the physician finds it distasteful to manage a practice (in the sense that the physician would pay someone else to perform management chores, and that amount would be greater than the physician would earn from any time thereby released). The pecuniary equivalent of any such distaste is netted out of "net professional income."

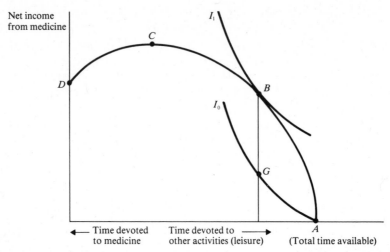

Fig. 4.1 Net professional income as a function of hours of medical practice. At point *A* the physician is devoting no hours to medicine, and at point *D* the physician is devoting all available time to medicine. The curve *ABCD* represents what the physician can earn practicing medicine. It is shown as turning down to the left of *C* on the presumption that the physician cannot effectively work all the time. The utility-maximizing physician chooses point *B*, where the locus *ABCD* is tangent to indifference curve I_1. Indifference curve I_0 shows the amount of income the physician must earn at each workload to be indifferent between practicing medicine and the next best alternative.

in that occupation. (Normal profits—the amount necessary to keep the entrepreneur in the industry—are included in standard cost curves.) That wage is shown as an indifference curve I_0 in Fig. 4.1. At any point on I_0 the physician is indifferent between not practicing medicine at all (point *A* is no time in medicine and no income from medicine) and receiving an amount of income with a corresponding medical workload shown on the indifference curve I_0. (The indifference curve thus reflects the opportunity cost of practicing medicine.)

Inspecting the figure, we can see that the assumption of profit maximization implies that the physician maximizes the difference between net income as shown on the curve *ABCD* and the implicit wage required to keep the physician practicing medicine as shown by indifference curve I_0. This difference is maximized when the slope of curve *ABCD* equals the slope of I_0. The greatest difference occurs at the same hours of work as the utility-maximizing hours of work if the slope of the indifference curves at a given number of hours is the same at various income levels (as drawn in the figure, because the slope of indifference curve I_1 at *B* is the same as I_0 at *G*). Restating this condition, the utility-maximizing number of hours will equal the profit-maximizing number of hours if the income elasticity for hours of work is zero, for then hours of work do not change with income. (If the income elasticity for work were negative, who would work more—a profit-maximizing physician or a utility-maximizing physician?

The force of the objection that physicians maximize utility and not profit therefore reduces to an empirical question: Is the income elasticity of physicians' hours of work near zero? If it is, the hours represented by B will be similar to the number of hours represented by G, and a theory that assumes profit maximization will yield approximately the same predictions as a theory that assumes utility maximization

Empirical evidence suggests that the income elasticity of physician hours of work is approximately zero. Sloan [2] estimates that an additional $2,000 in annual income in 1970 would reduce physician hours of work by around 1 percent, and the 1-percent figure is statistically indistinguishable from no effect at all. Hence it does not really matter for predictive purposes that the physician maximizes utility rather than net income, assuming that utility is a function of net income and leisure; the predictions of interest are to a first approximation identical under either assumption.

An important general lesson in this example is that a theory can make "unrealistic" assumptions (in this case profit maximization) but still yield valid predictions. Thus a theory should not be rejected simply because its assumptions are unrealistic or even known to be wrong. In fact, all theory must be unrealistic to some degree, because theory attempts to predict the future based on past experience. Because the future is never exactly like the past in every detail, the assumptions we make for predictive purposes (i.e., that the circumstances we know something about will hold in the future) will always be somewhat in error. The issue is whether the amount of error is important or inconsequential, and that is both a logical question (would different assumptions produce different predictions?) and an empirical question (is the amount of any difference quantitatively important?).

WHAT ARE THE CONSEQUENCES OF RESTRICTING ENTRY?

A second objection to applying the idealized market model to medical care is the lack of free entry. Physicians must obtain a license to practice, and in order to do so they must graduate from a medical school. As premedical students know all too well, the number of medical school places falls considerably short of the number of students who wish to attend. Students who are not admitted have the options of attending medical school abroad or not practicing medicine, but entry is hardly free.

Fortunately, economists have a good deal of practice analyzing markets without free entry, and so this objection is relatively easy to meet. Suppose first that the firms (physicians) in the industry compete much as perfectly competitive firms, but that certain barriers limit the number of firms in the industry. In such a situation, existing firms may be earning rents, as shown by the vertical distance *BG* in Fig. 4.1. (Rent is a payment to a firm above that necessary to keep it in the industry.) If entry were free, the *marginal* firm would earn no rent; that is, the marginal would-be physician would be indifferent between pursuing medicine and the next most attractive occupation. (Points *B* and *G* would coincide.) If rent is being earned, price will be higher than if entry were free, and price will be determined by demand. (If demand increases, other things being equal, price will rise.) In many instances the rent will not ultimately accrue to those who gain admittance to an industry, because to obtain the privilege to enter they will have paid a price that effectively appropriates the rent. (For example, if taxicab medallions are required to operate a cab, the purchase price of a medallion will reflect the rent that can be earned.) Premedical students may wish to speculate on whether the "rat race" to gain admission to medical school has the effect of driving the return from a career in medicine down to a competitive rate.

An alternative assumption is that firms in the industry are not perfectly competitive. Suppose, for example, that each physician in the local area is a monopolist who faces a downward-sloping demand curve. In this case the standard theory of monopoly applies. However, such an assumption lessens the issue of free entry into medicine because there are already 300,000 physicians. If each of them is a monopolist in a local area, additional physicians are not likely to change the situation.

A middle ground between pure monopoly and pure competition is so-called imperfect or monopolistic competition. In this case each firm faces a downward-sloping demand curve, but the firms are interdependent; a given firm's actions have a noticeable impact on the other firms, and they respond to those actions. Moreover, the firm takes account of the response by the others in formulating its own actions. Analysis of such cases is difficult, and will not be discussed here, except to note that lowering barriers to entry imposed by licensure is not likely to transform monopolistic competition to pure competition. In sum, the economist's models can accomodate barriers to entry.

CONSUMER IGNORANCE

Economic theory assumes that the consumer has well-defined preferences, but some maintain that there are instances in which the consumer's preferences should not be satisfied. Often the justification for not honoring the consumer's preferences is consumer ignorance. It is argued that if the consumer knew more, choices would be different. For example, if the consumer knew as much about disease as the physician, there might be little non-compliance with physician directives, such as not taking prescribed medicines. Presumed ignorance has on occasion led society not to honor preferences—children are not allowed to contract, nor are inmates of mental hospitals. One is not allowed to sell oneself into slavery. But these are rather extreme cases; generally Western democracies have accorded their citizens the right to choose what to consume, including the right to make mistakes.

Against this background, what can be said about consumer ignorance and medicine? Fortunately, consumer ignorance is not much of an issue with respect to positive economics, the study of what is. For example, one can measure the responsiveness of demand to insurance as we did in Chapter 2, and for purposes of prediction all one must assume is that over time consumer knowledge remains roughly constant. Of course, if consumers became much more (or much less) knowledgeable, one's predictions might miss rather badly, but such change does not seem likely.

The difficult issue arises with respect to normative economics, the study of what should be. Here one can argue that the consumer's ignorance makes possible manipulation by the physician (or other provider) to the consumer's detriment. We shall take up the issue of manipulation in the next section; here it suffices to point out that the mere demonstration of consumer manipulation does not in itself justify public sector intervention to alter the market outcome. Rather than comparing the outcome to an idealized intervention, one must assess actual outcomes when the public sector does or does not intervene. This issue will be a major focus in Chapter 6.

Thus, for the purposes of Chapter 2 and this chapter, which are primarily concerned with understanding existing phenomena, consumer ignorance is of little consequence. For the purpose of Chapter 6, which is concerned with what should be, consumer ignorance is of considerable consequence. Further discussion of this issue can be found in that chapter.

DO PHYSICIANS CREATE THEIR OWN DEMAND?

Much of the price mechanism's appeal is the sovereignty of the consumer; the consumer can direct the flow of recources in the economy through dollar "votes." The desirability of consumer sovereignty assumes that consumers have well-defined tastes for goods and services. When applied to medical care, this assumption is often questioned. It is argued that the physician can manipulate the consumer and create demand for physician services. For several years the ability of the physician to create demand has been debated (for example, [3, 4, 5]). We will not settle the debate here, although we shall see that the underlying issues are more subtle than the title of this subsection indicates.

The discussion of demand creation often takes place in the context of changing the numbers of physicians. At one extreme are those who believe that entry into medicine has been artificially constrained, and that consumers' welfare would be improved by adding more physicians [6]. Behind this view of the world lies the assumption that the medical marketplace functions approximately like a competitive marketplace, except that entry into it has been restricted by the profession. Thus, more physicians will overcome the pernicious effects of professional prophylaxis. In this view, adding physicians would raise the quantity of medical services, lower their price, and most importantly reallocate resources toward medicine.

At the other extreme are those who believe that the physician possesses almost unlimited ability to induce demand for services. Behind this view of the world lies the assumption that the medical marketplace is not competitive, and that additional physicians will merely create work for themselves by recommending needless operations, performing more tests, and advising consumers to return for unnecessary observation ([3, 5, 7, 8]; for contrary evidence, see [9]). Those of this persuasion agree that adding physicians will raise the quantity of medical services, but believe that this reallocation of resources toward medicine is undesirable. [4]

A critical question in this debate is whether increasing the supply of medical services can create demand. In support of this proposition it is pointed out that areas with more physicians utilize more physician services, areas with more hospital beds use more hospital services, and so forth. Unfortunately for the pursuit of knowledge, this fact does not show that supply creates its own demand.

Recall what happens when the supply of a good increases in a competitive market. Consider the wheat market, and suppose that the weather has been much better than in the previous year. Then we can expect the supply curve to shift rightward. Figure 4.2 shows a shift from AB to CD, a rise in the quantity of wheat consumed from q_0 to q_1, and a fall in the price from P_0 to P_1. Those who believe the medical marketplace is competitive believe that it functions like the wheat market.

Return now to the observed positive association between the supply of physicians and hospitals and the quantity of medical services consumed. Figure 4.2 makes clear that such an association is quite consistent with the competitive model, because in a competitive marketplace there is a positive correlation between shifts in the supply schedule and amount consumed. (What is the one exception?) Hence, showing that there are more medical services consumed in areas with large numbers of physicians and hospital beds does not prove that physicians (much less beds!) can create their own demand.

---

4 Occasionally, the estimates of the previous chapter are cited to show that medical services could be expanded more efficiently by adding paramedical personnel instead of physicians.

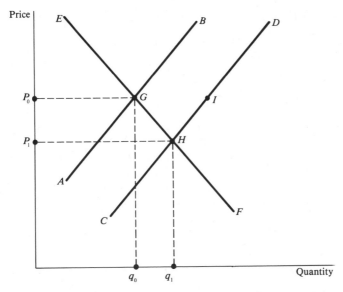

Fig. 4.2 A competitive equilibrium. In a competitive marketplace an increase in the supply of a good causes price to fall and quantity consumed to rise.

A more sophisticated formulation of this argument takes cognizance of the downward-sloping demand curve. This formulation argues that in a competitive market (in which supply did not create demand), additional supply (physicians or beds) would be associated with additional consumption, but the increase in consumption would not equal the full increase in supply because demand is not perfectly elastic. Thus, in Fig. 4.2, the rise in consumption from q_0 to q_1 is less than the shift in supply (from G to I). Because we know the demand curve for medical care slopes down, goes the argument, we can test whether supply creates its own demand by seeing if utilization rises by an amount equal to the rise in supply. If it does, this would be evidence against the competitive model and for the hypothesis that supply creates its own demand. Unfortunately, there is also a problem with this test.

In the wheat market the buyer pays the seller directly. As we have seen, the medical care sector frequently interposes another party between the buyer and the seller; this "third" party (which may be an insurance company or the state) pays the seller on behalf of the buyer. This does create difficulties for the competitive model, as we shall show in the next section. But it also means that the test described in the preceding paragraph cannot necessarily serve as a test of whether supply creates its own demand.

To see why, suppose that there is a national health plan in which patients pay little or nothing for medical services; the state supplies (or pays for) the services (for example, the British National Health Service). In that case demand and supply curves for hospital beds might look like those illustrated in Fig. 4.3, in which the equilibrium price is at p_0, but the price to the consumer is at p_c (p_c might be zero). Because the physician is so instrumental in the utilization of hospital services, we shall henceforth speak of the consumer/physician team as the demander. At the price p_c consumer/physician team desires to purchase the quantity on the demand curve denoted by M. However, the state does not supply this much; rather, it pays an amount equal to the difference between p_s and p_c (if p_c is zero, then the state's payment is p_s), and suppliers produce an amount equal to q_0. (Why?) The difference between q_0 and M represents excess demand, an amount the consumer/physician team wants to buy but that is not available. In a competitive market price would rise to p_0. Because the state keeps the monetary price at p_c, nonprice rationing will arise (for example, queues) to determine who receives the services available. (Recall the queues in Montreal referred to in Chapter 2.)

Now suppose the state adds more hospital beds, so that the supply curve shifts rightward. Supply rises from q_0 to q_1, as does the amount consumed. Note that in this case, unlike that diagrammed in Fig. 4.2, the amount consumed rises by the *entire* amount of the increase in supply. Thus, if prices are below market clearing prices, showing that consumption of services rises equally with supply does not prove that supply creates

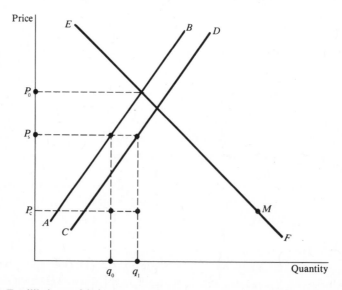

Fig. 4.3 Equilibrium with insurance coverage. In the presence of insurance there may be nonprice rationing of services.

demand. In effect, prices do not have to fall to induce the consumer/ physician team to purchase more of the good when its supply increases; the team already wants more of the good at the existing price than is available. In the presence of excess demand, a test of demand creation based on whether demand rises by the entire amount of the supply increase fails.

All this may sound rather abstract and foreign to one convinced that physicians create their own demand. An image that comes to mind, for example, is the surgeon's advising the patient that surgery is necessary, when in fact the indications are questionable. Some believe that this becomes more prevalent when there are additional surgeons. This notion too can be represented with our supply and demand curve apparatus. Figure 4.4 shows an increase in supply (the shift from *AB* to *CD*), and a corresponding increase in demand that is assumed to occur because the additional supply (say of physicians) creates demand (the demand curve shifts outward from *EF* to *GH*). Because both supply and demand curves shift out, quantity consumed rises from q_0 to q_1; however, whether price rises or falls depends on the relative magnitude of the shifts in the supply and demand curves. As drawn, price rises from p_0 to p_1, but if the shift in the demand curve is small relative to the shift in the supply curve, price would fall.

Such reasoning has formed the basis of another proposed test of whether supply creates its own demand, namely whether greater supply (typically more physicians per person) is associated with higher or lower

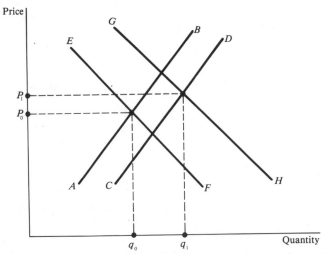

Fig. 4.4 Supply creates its own demand. An increase in supply is shown along with an increase in demand. Under these circumstances, the quantity consumed rises and price may rise or fall, depending on elasticities of demand and supply and the amount of the shifts in the demand and supply schedules.

prices for medical services. Figure 4.2 shows that in a competitive market, price would fall if supply were increased, whereas Fig. 4.4 shows that if supply affected demand, price might increase or decrease. Hence, the argument goes, if prices are observed to increase with increasing supply, one can reject the competitive model and accept the hypothesis that supply creates its own demand.

Empirical studies of this matter are conflicting, but there is some evidence that the price of a physician visit does rise with additional physicians. Suppose this evidence were correct; would that constitute grounds for rejecting the competitive model? Unfortunately, the test based on the association between price and physician supply also has an Achilles heel, having to do with the nature of the product. Recall that analysis of a competitive market assumes a fixed and homogeneous product. But physicians in areas with greater concentration of physicians spend more time with their patients and patients in such areas spend less time waiting for their physicians [10, 11]. More time with the physician and less waiting time are both desirable characteristics that lead to more physician time per visit. In a competitive market, visits using more physician time would be more expensive. As a result, even if the market were competitive, there could be a positive relationship between the physician/population ratio and the price of a (non-homogeneous) physician visit. The test of demand creation based on physician prices also fails.

In the end the emperor has no clothes; no one has yet specified a method for unambiguously testing whether supply creates its own demand. In principle, one could use a test based on price if the characteristics of the product (visit) could be held constant, but in practice that is hard to do (and a skeptic can always wonder whether *all* the characteristics of the product have in fact been held constant).

Such a conclusion is disappointing, and a frustrated reader might conclude that Burke was redundant in commenting that the age of economists and sophisters had succeeded. After all, one might argue, isn't it obvious that physicians influence demand for their services? One merely has to think back to one's last visit to the physician. Did not the physician make recommendations about treatment that (probably) were followed? Thus, can we not conclude that the physician influences demand?

The answer to this question is probably yes, but the question is not germane to the debates over the numbers of physicians or the role of the consumer. The underlying issues are more subtle. In the debate over the appropriate number of physicians, the question is not whether the physician influences or creates demand, but whether the amount of influence depends on the number of physicians. In other words, the real issue is whether the physician has *unexploited* ability to create demand, and whether the degree to which the physician exploits that ability varies with the number of physicians in the area. In the debate over whether the physician manipulates the consumer in a manner not in the consumer's interest, the real issue is whether the physician acts only in the patient's best interests (that is, acts as the patient's agent). The answers to these questions cannot be found by thinking back on one's last physician visit.[5]

Thus we reach an impasse. A simple empirical test has not yet been devised of whether physicians have unexploited ability to create demand. As a result, the objection to the competitive model that supply (physicians) creates its own demand can be neither ruled out nor confirmed on the basis of empirical data. In such circumstances the way to proceed depends on whether one is asking positive or normative questions.

When in the realm of positive economics, one can continue to use the competitive model. To modify that model in ways that allow the physician to manipulate demand is certainly possible, but if it does not produce conclusions that differ from the simpler competitive model, why bother? (This follows from a general scientific principle known as Occam's Razor; if a complicated model and a simple model both produce the same predictions, one should prefer the simple model.) Of course, if the results of a modified model did differ from the competitive model, then one would examine actual data to determine which model was consistent with them.

For normative purposes the matter is different, because consumer sovereignty presumes that consumer demands should be satisfied. But if the consumer is but jelly in the hands of the physician, there can be no presumption that the demands of the consumer/physician team should be satisfied. Further discussion of consumer sovereignty is deferred to the last chapter. In the remaining part of this chapter, we consider an objection to the competitive model even as a tool of positive economics.

WHAT IS THE BASIS FOR PRICE COMPETITION IN AN INSURED MARKET?

In the competitive model consumers are assumed to maximize their utility. As a result, they have an incentive to search for the lowest cost supplier of a good or service, for if they can find the lowest cost supplier, they will have more money to purchase other goods and services (and so will be able to increase their utility). If information about prices and product quality were costless to obtain, prices would be approximately identical among all suppliers, for no utility-maximizing consumer would patronize a supplier who

---

5 An interesting study [12] of surgery rates among physicians and their families compared with rates among attorneys found no significant difference, suggesting that in this case physicians were acting as the patient's agent.

charged more than the lowest cost.[6] Of course, information about suppliers is costly to obtain (restrictions on advertising make it more costly), and so consumers may not know that any given supplier is in fact the lowest-cost supplier. Moreover, it may not pay consumers to invest time and effort to find out which supplier is the lowest cost. (How many stores do you visit to ascertain the price of pencils?) The utility-maximizing consumer will trade off the cost of additional search for the lowest-cost supplier against the expected savings from such search. As a result of incomplete search, a competitive market will exhibit price dispersion.

Nonetheless, each seller in a competitive marketplace (including those who are not least cost) can expect to lose customers if that seller raises price; fewer of those consumers who search will patronize the seller with a higher price, and some customers who did not search may be motivated to begin searching when price rises. Similarly, a monopolist who raises price can expect to lose business, as consumers substitute other products and move back up their demand curves; indeed, a profit-maximizing monopolist by definition seeks that price at which any further increase reduces profits. Hence, in both monopolistic and competitive industries, market forces exist that determine price and give suppliers incentives not to raise price above a certain point. In this section we show that this mechanism has partially broken down in the medical care market.

The structure of present health insurance policies causes the breakdown of price competition. Consider a typical hospital group insurance plan. The monthly premium is the same for all members of the group (save for differences in family structure), and the insurance will pay the entire bill for any hospitalization. But precisely because insurance pays, the consumer/physician team has no incentive to find the lowest-cost hospital; all members of the group will share any extra costs of the hospitalization, and the consumer's own premium will be negligibly affected. If any search takes place, it will be for the hospital that provides the best product without reference to cost.

Some polices do have a coinsurance rate, although rarely does the coinsurance rate exceed 25 percent, and frequently it is less. Suppose there is a 25-percent coinsurance rate. Then, if the consumer/physician team can find a lower-cost supplier, the consumer will receive $1 out of every $4 saved. Such savings give some incentive to search for a lower-cost supplier. But recall that the maximizing consumer balances the cost of additional

---

6 Differentials among suppliers might appear because of transportation costs. Also, all consumers do not have to maximize utility to drive high-cost suppliers out of business; if most consumers maximize utility and patronize only the lowest-cost supplier, while other nonmaximizing consumers distribute themselves at random among suppliers, the higher-cost supplier may not receive enough business to survive.

search against the expected savings from such search. If 75 percent or more of the savings accrue to the insurance company, the scales are tipped rather heavily toward less search.

In fact, around 92 percent of all hospital bills are now paid for by an insurance company or by the government. An unknown amount of the remaining 8 percent (but probably a substantial portion of it) goes for an initial deductible that is exceeded during the stay. (You can test your understanding of Chapter 2 by showing that such a deductible will not materially affect choice of hospital.) Another part of the remaining 8 percent finances certain particular services that are less well insured but constitute a separate market (most notably maternity services). As a result, the hospital marketplace for most services approximates virtually full insurance.

Consider now the incentives facing the decisionmaker in the hospital.[7] Suppose the decisionmaker is deciding whether to purchase a new machine or whether to grant the hospital's employees a wage increase. In a competitive industry factors are hired until their marginal revenue product equals their marginal factor cost. An equilibrium exists because the marginal revenue product falls as more of the factor is hired, while the marginal factor price is constant or rises. (Marginal revenue product falls because there is a fixed product price facing the firm, and additional units of the factor are assumed to be less productive than the initial units.)

The hospital decisionmaker does not operate in a competitive industry. Most customers (patients) are covered by insurance that will either reimburse the hospital directly for costs (government programs and Blue Cross-Blue Shield) or reimburse the patient for the hospital's charges (commercial insurance companies). (Reimbursement of costs usually means that if an expenditure is legitimately related to patient care, it will be paid.) Given reimbursement of costs or charges, there is little incentive not to add the machine or raise wages. Some public relations problems may arise, but unlike higher prices in other industries, the higher price of hospital care will not cause a fully insured patient/physician team to seek care at another hospital, to refrain from entering the hospital, or to use fewer services once hospitalized. In effect, the hospital decisionmaker receives a signal from the market to add factors until their marginal product is zero. (Does this imply that in matters of health society wants only the best?) Furthermore, squeezing more production out of given resources yields the hospital little reward because consumer/physician teams are not motivated to search for efficient suppliers. This is a type of market failure.

Notice, however, that insuring a few consumers has different effects from insuring most consumers. (There is a fallacy of composition.) If no

---

7 The exact identity of "the decisionmaker" in the hospital is discussed in the Appendix of this chapter.

one else were insured, a few consumers could be insured and the insurance company could reimburse the hospital at the rate that noninsured consumers paid for services. In fact, a phrase in many health insurance policies (including Medicare) states that the insurer will pay the provider at a usual, customary, or reasonable rate. If almost no consumers were insured (and the medical marketplace were otherwise competitive), the usual, customary, or reasonable rate could be defined as the competitive price, and that price would be observable from market transactions.

But the situation changes drastically when virtually everyone is insured. In that case the provider need not take account of noninsured individuals (that is, the market for services to noninsured individuals is very small); consequently, the rates charged noninsured individuals are not competitively established prices. The phrase usual, customary, and reasonable then changes meaning, and in practice does not refer to the rates charged noninsured individuals, but rather the rates charged other insured individuals and rates charged by other providers. If all providers charge the same amount and all raise their prices 15 percent per year, there is little or no resistance from the insurance company.

One other possible restraint on providers may occur to some readers. While an increase in rates will not drive a fully insured consumer/ physician team to another hospital, it will increase the premiums that all privately insured consumers pay. It is possible theoretically that the higher premiums (caused by the higher medical care prices) would lead consumers to purchase less insurance. If so, the market could be self-correcting; higher prices would lead to less insurance, which in turn would act as a force for lower prices. Unfortunately, it is also possible that higher medical care prices would make consumers want insurance even more than before. Empirically, the forces leading consumers to purchase more insurance as prices go up roughly cancel the forces leading them to purchase less (or may be somewhat stronger). That 92 percent of expenditures for hospital services are covered despite persistently large rates of inflation (see Table 4.1) indicates that consumers do not markedly reduce their purchases of insurance as medical care prices rise.

One other important influence of insurance deserves mention—its effects on new products. In a competitive industry those engaged in research and development of new products are on notice that cost is a relevant consideration; if the new product is sufficiently expensive, consumers may not be willing to pay for it. With the present structure of hospital insurance, those engaged in research and development for hospital services receive a different kind of signal—there will be a buyer for virtually any new product with a positive marginal product. This simply extends to changes in technology the previous argument that there is an incentive to employ any factor until its marginal product is zero. Hence the structure of insurance

Table 4.1 Percentage increases in price and insurance coverage for four medical services, 1949–1975

Service	Average annual percentage price increase	Average percentage of bill covered by third party during this period
Hospital	8.66	82.3
Physician	4.09	38.7
Dentist	3.52	3.3
Drug	0.94	4.4
Overall consumer price index	2.83	—

Source: Newhouse [13].

also induces a part of the costly technological change that we observe in medical care.

Because hospital services have been well insured for many years, it is not surprising that hospital prices have shown extraordinarily large rates of increase for a long time. Table 4.1 lists the average insurance coverage and the average rates of price increase for four medical services in the 1949–1975 period. Hospital services show the fastest rate of price increase, while drugs show the least. Analysis of year-to-year price changes for these four services shows that the rate of increase of hospital prices is well above what might be predicted from a competitive model [13]. The marketplace for hospital services, as presently structured, appears to have failed, and so a competitive supply curve is not well defined. What might be done about this failure is the subject of Chapter 6.

CONCLUSION

The most important feature of the medical care marketplace from the vantage point of economics is that the structure of existing health insurance has severely abridged price competition. There is little or no basis for price competition when insurance simply reimburses costs (or charges). Not only does the consumer/physician team face incentives to demand the best, they are not even motivated to seek care from an efficient supplier of the best! The nature of the supply curve for hospitals is at the moment an open question.

Consumer ignorance of medical care technology raises troublesome problems for a normative analysis of medical care, but is of less consequence for positive analysis that asks questions such as: What is the effect on demand of lowering the coinsurance rate? What is the effect on employ-ment of aides of raising their wage rate? Answers to such questions assume that the amount of ignorance is roughly constant over time and thus can be ignored. Restrictions on entry and providers' interest in leisure as well as income cause no real difficulty for traditional economic models. Although the simplest models may need modification when such phenomena are pre-sent, the nature of these modifications is well understood and widely agreed upon.

REFERENCES

1. Tibor Scitovsky. "A Note on Profit Maximization and Its Implications." *Review of Economic Studies,* Vol. 11: 57–60, 1943. Reprinted in *Readings in Price Theory,* edited by George Stigler and Kenneth Boulding. Chicago: Irwin, 1952.

2. Frank A. Sloan. "Physician Supply Behavior in the Short Run." *Industrial and Labor Relations Review* 28, No. 4: 549–569 (July 1975).

3. Robert G. Evans. "Supplier-Induced Demand: Some Empirical Evidence and Implications." In *The Economics of Health and Medical Care: Proceedings of a Conference Held by the International Economic Association at Tokyo,* edited by Mark Perlman. London: Macmillan, 1974.

4. Frank A. Sloan and Roger Feldman. "Monopolistic Elements in the Market for Physicians' Services." Paper given at a Federal Trade Commission Conference on Competition in the Health Care Sector: Past, Present, and Future, Washington, June 1977.

5. Uwe E. Reinhardt. "Parkinson's Law and the Demand for Physicians' Services: Comment on the Paper Presented by Sloan and Feldman at the Federal Trade Commission Conference, 1977." (See reference 4.)

6. Reuben A. Kessel. "Higher Education and the Nation's Health: A Review of the Carnegie Commission Report on Medical Education." *Journal of Law and Economics* 15, No. 1: 115–128 (April 1972).

7. Charles E. Lewis. "Variations in the Incidence of Surgery." *New England Journal of Medicine* 281, No. 16: 880–884 (16 October, 1969).

8. John Wennberg and Alan Gittelsohn. "Small Area Variations in Health Care Delivery." *Science* 182: 1102–1108 (14 December, 1973).

9. Noralou P. Roos, Leslie L. Roos, Jr., and Paul D. Henteleff. "Elective Surgical Rates—Do High Rates Mean Lower Standards?" *New England Journal of Medicine* 297, No. 7: 360–365 (18 August, 1977).

10. Frank A. Sloan and John Lorant. "The Allocation of Physicians' Services: Evidence on Length-of-Visit." *Quarterly Review of Economics and Business* 16, No. 3: 85–103 (Autumn 1976).

11. Frank A. Sloan and John Lorant. "The Role of Waiting Time: Evidence from Physicians' Practices." *Journal of Business,* forthcoming.

12. John P. Bunker and Byron William Brown, Jr. "The Physician-Patient as an Informed Consumer of Surgical Services." *New England Journal of Medicine* 290, No. 19: 1051–1055 (9 May, 1974).

13. Joseph P. Newhouse. "The Erosion of the Medical Marketplace." Santa Monica: The Rand Corporation, R-2141-HEW, 1977.

Appendix to Chapter 4 How Do Hospitals Make Choices

Hospital care is the most expensive portion of medical care; including inpatient physician fees, over half of all medical care dollars are spent in the hospital [1]. Most hospitals are not for profit.[1] Because standard economic theory assumes that firms maximize profits, it cannot be straightforwardly applied to hospital behavior.

The importance of hospitals justifies discussion of their behavior as firms, but I have relegated this material to an Appendix because of the unsatisfactory state of the literature.[2] The numerous theories of hospital behavior have generated few testable hypotheses, and little actual testing has occurred, making discrimination among the various theories difficult.

Theories of nonprofit hospital behavior have focused on two possible differences from perfectly competitive, profit-maximizing firms: (1) whether hospitals minimize the cost of production for a given output mix; and (2) whether hospitals produce different products or different quantities than a perfectly competitive firm. Chapter 6 demonstrates that the perfectly competitive firm produces efficiently; most of the literature assumes that if the nonprofit firm differs, it is inefficient. I shall discuss this assumption at the conclusion of the Appendix; for now I accept it.

No one has estimated the precise magnitude of any inefficiencies attributable to the tax and legal advantages conferred on the nonprofit hospital, but Manning has concluded that they are small [7]. Such a conclusion is

---

1 Nonprofit hospitals accounted for over two-thirds of all admissions to short-term general and other special hospitals in 1976 [2].
2 A very complete review of the literature can be found in [3]; other reviews are in [4], [5], [6].

plausible, because the advantages of nonprofit status are not so great as to preclude competition from for-profit hospitals.[3]

Although inefficiency from nonprofit status per se may be small, we saw in the last section of this chapter that the product market facing all hospitals differs markedly from that of a perfectly competitive firm and may induce substantial inefficiencies. Hospitals that do not minimize cost are not necessarily driven out of existence by consumers taking their business elsewhere. Because the permissive product market appears to allow the hospital some discretion, the incentives of decisionmakers at nonprofit hospitals deserve consideration.

DO HOSPITALS MINIMIZE COSTS?

Some theories of the nonprofit hospital suggest it does not minimize cost. For the most part these theories emphasize the role of slack [8,9].[4] *Slack* represents an expenditure that management desires for its own sake or for prestige; extra thick carpets in the administrator's office are an example. Managements of all firms are hypothesized to desire slack; in the for-profit sector, however, the competitiveness of the product market restrains the amount of slack.

In addition to the weakness of competitive forces in the hospital market, certain features of nonprofit institutions may increase the scope for slack. Tax and legal advantages have already been mentioned. Furthermore, Clarkson [12] has suggested that decisionmakers at nonprofit hospitals do not have exclusive rights to the benefits (profits) produced by the enterprise; as a result, he infers that managerial actions will emphasize current benefits to the manager (slack) at the expense of future benefits to the organization. If slack could be measured, the importance of nonprofit status relative to the product market in explaining slack at hospitals could be ascertained by comparing hospitals with other private nonprofit institutions (for example, private universities; the amount of endowment should be controlled for); if the amount of slack was much greater at hospitals, one could infer that product market differences were important. In the absence of data, the amount and etiology of slack remain speculative.

Pauly and Redisch [13] and Manning [7] have developed a second cause of inefficient hospital production. They emphasize the role of the physician in making hospital decisions; Pauly and Redisch assume hospital decisions are made by physicians to maximize their income, and patients demand hos-

---

3 Ten percent of the admissions to private short-term general and other special hospitals occur in for-profit hospitals [2].

4 The term *slack* comes from [10]; see also [11].

pital and physician services jointly. If patients paid less for hospital services, they would be willing to pay more for physician services. Hence, physician income in the aggregate would be maximized if hospital costs were minimized, but cost minimization requires that all physicians act as a single decisionmaker, which is difficult.

Individual physicians control the application of hospital inputs to specific patients under their care, and additional hospital inputs may enhance the physician's income. Because the full costs of the inputs may be spread over all patients, the individual physician has an incentive to overorder inputs (relative to the situation where the entire medical staff acts as one decisionmaker). For example, suppose nurses' services are part of the daily rate charged all hospital patients, and a physician can effectively argue for more nurses on a particular unit. The additional nurses may increase the productivity and income of the physician, but their cost will be borne by all hospital patients, not just the patients of that physician. Readers may wish to speculate whether faculties play a role at universities similar to physicians at a hospital.

Pauly and Redisch and Manning predict that any inefficiency from overordering of inputs will be greater, the greater the size of the hospital. At smaller hospitals physicians can monitor each other's behavior more easily and minimize any tendency to overorder (that is, it is easier for a small group to act as a single decisionmaker). Manning [7] finds some support for this hypothesis.[5]

CHOOSING THE WRONG PRODUCTS

The hospital may be inefficient in its selection of products for the same reason that it may use slack inputs; namely, a benefit accrues to the firm's management that does not accrue in similar measure to the community [14, 15, 16]. The ability to treat individuals with a certain disease, or to care for patients in a particular ("high quality") fashion, may be more highly valued by the hospital's administrator, trustees, and physician staff than by the community, especially if the community already can obtain that particular treatment (the product) at another hospital.

The existence of tax and legal benefits allows the nonprofit hospital to subsidize the production of certain products or quality levels that a for-profit firm would not undertake. Some empirical evidence supports the hypothesis that nonprofit institutions provide a higher quality product than for-profit institutions, as quality is conventionally measured. More non-

---

5 Manning is one of the few who attempts empirical tests of his hypotheses. Unfortunately, all of his empirical results are suspect because data were not available to him to control for differences in types of cases treated across hospitals.

profit hospitals than for-profit hospitals are accredited, and more nonprofit nursing homes have a registered nurse as the top skill level rather than a licensed practical nurse (or neither a registered nurse nor a licensed practical nurse) [16]. The capacity to treat patients requiring open-heart surgery (which carries professional prestige) appears excessive; a presidential commission in the mid-1960s found that 30 percent of the hospitals equipped to perform open-heart surgery had no cases in the year under study [16]. The increase in "quality" uses resources that the community might have preferred to use elsewhere, but no researcher has made a comprehensive estimate of the costs of possible selection of wrong products.

DOES DIVERGENCE FROM PERFECT COMPETITION REALLY REPRESENT INEFFICIENCY?

Harris has recently suggested that the standard of perfect competition may not be useful for judging the efficiency of hospitals (both nonprofit and for-profit) [17]. He views the hospital as two firms in one, each firm having its own managers, objectives, and pricing strategies. The medical staff is one firm; it could also be characterized as a demand division, deciding whether a patient is admitted, which tests are ordered, and whether an operation is performed. The hospital administration is the other firm, and it could be characterized as a supply division, providing certain services (nursing, laboratory, X-ray) to the medical staff.

Each physician on the medical staff wishes services to be available if that physician's patient should require them. Demand at the hospital fluctuates randomly (on certain days the hospital is more crowded), but the price system cannot readily be used to allocate resources when capacity is stressed.[6] In lieu of the price system, a system of informal rules has developed to allocate resources. The rules function somewhat like an honor system; for example, physicians classify their laboratory test orders as routine and "stat"; the latter take priority. When the hospital nears capacity, the rules tend to break down as physicians hoard resources on behalf of their patients. For example, a high proportion of lab test orders may become stat.

Harris argues that some unused capacity is a necessary price to pay to keep the system of informal rules from breaking down, that is, to facilitate accommodation within the physician staff and between the two firms within the hospital. But such unused capacity can be described as excess only when

---

6 Harris's example is that "it would be intolerable for Dr. A and Dr. B to haggle over the market clearing price of, say, one available intensive care bed which was immediately needed by both of their patients." Analytically, demand is highly inelastic and decisions must often be made quickly by the doctor acting as an agent. In many cases both patients will be fully insured.

judged against an ideal that is probably unattainable, a "single-firm" hospital. For even if physicians were both demanders and suppliers, as in a prepaid group practice that owns its own hospital, the incentive remains for individual physicians to hoard as capacity is approached. (Note the similarity with the Pauly-Redisch and Manning argument that individual physicians may not act in their best interest as a group.) If a single-firm hospital is impossible, at least some of the hospital's alleged inefficiencies may be inescapable; there could be little scope for more efficient production. Such a hypothesis could be tested if the product market became more competitive (see Chapter 6). Until then the possible magnitude of inefficiencies must remain conjectural.

A policy postscript emerges from the "two-firm" nature of the hospital. Although we will analyze regulation in Chapter 6, it is relevant to point out here that proposed controls on hospital revenues (so-called cost containment) assume a single decisionmaker at the hospital. In fact, individual physicians tend to control the quantity of services delivered, while the administrator controls their unit price. For a single decisionmaker (for example, the hospital administrator) to ensure operation within a given budget would require control of physician decisions on individual patient management. Only very crude mechanisms for exerting such control now exist, and undoubtedly more powerful controls would have to be established if such regulation took effect. How such controls would operate is unknown, and therefore whether they would prove beneficial on balance is unknown. Moreover, both proposed controls on hospital revenues and existing regulation of hospital capital investment (Certificate-of-Need laws) have reduction in hospital capacity as an objective. Harris predicts that if regulation of either revenues or investment markedly reduces capacity, the system of informal rules governing physician behavior could break down to the patient's detriment.

REFERENCES

1. Joseph P. Newhouse, Charles E. Phelps, and William B. Schwartz. "Policy Options and the Impact of National Health Insurance." *New England Journal of Medicine* 290, No. 24: 1345–1359 (13 June, 1974).

2. American Hospital Association. *AHA Guide to the Health Care Field, 1977 Edition*. Chicago: The Association, 1977.

3. Sylvester E. Berki. *Hospital Economics*. Lexington, Mass.: D. C. Heath, 1972.

4. Karen Davis. "Economic Theories of Behavior in Nonprofit Private Hospitals." *Economic and Business Bulletin* 24, No. 2: 1–13 (Winter 1972).

5. Martin S. Feldstein. "Econometric Studies of Health Economics." In *Frontiers of Quantitative Economics, II*, edited by Michael Intriligator and David Kendrick. Amsterdam: North Holland, 1974.

6. Philip Jacobs. "A Survey of Economic Models of Hospitals." *Inquiry* 11, No. 2: 83–97 (June 1974).

7. Willard G. Manning, Jr. "Comparable Efficiency in Short-Term General Hospitals." Stanford University Center for Research in Economic Growth, Research Memorandum 154, 1973.

8. Robert G. Evans. "'Behavioral' Cost Functions for Hospitals." *Canadian Journal of Economics* 4, No. 2: 198–215 (May 1971).

9. Paul B. Ginsburg. "Regulating the Price of Hospital Care." Paper prepared for the Regulatory Reform Conference, American Enterprise Institute, Washington, 1975.

10. R. M. Cyert and J. G. March. *A Behavioral Theory of the Firm*. Englewood Cliffs, N. J.: Prentice-Hall, 1963.

11. Oliver E. Williamson. *The Economics of Discretionary Behavior: Managerial Objectives in a Theory of the Firm*. Chicago: Markham, 1967.

12. Kenneth W. Clarkson. "Some Implications of Property Rights in Hospital Management." *Journal of Law and Economics* 15, No. 2: 363–384 (October 1972).

13. Mark Pauly and Michael Redisch. "The Not-For-Profit Hospital as a Physicians' Cooperative." *American Economic Review* 63, No. 1: 87–99 (March 1973).

14. Martin S. Feldstein. "Hospital Cost Inflation: A Study of Nonprofit Price Dynamics." *American Economic Review* 61, No. 5: 853–872 (December 1971).

15. Maw Lin Lee. "A Conspicuous Production Theory of Hospital Behavior." *Southern Economic Journal* 38, No. 1: 48–59 (July 1971).

16. Joseph P. Newhouse. "Toward a Theory of Nonprofit Institutions: An Economic Model of a Hospital." *American Economic Review* 60, No. 1: 64–74 (March 1971).

17. Jeffrey Harris. "The Internal Organization of Hospitals: Some Economic Implications." *The Bell Journal of Economics* 8, No. 2: 467–482 (Autumn 1977).

The Output of the Medical Care Delivery System 5

Thus far we have described the product of the medical care system as physician visits, hospital days, and the like. For example, we measured the marginal product of aides in units of physician visits (Fig. 3.3). But is one interested in such outputs?

Some argue that the delivery system really produces health, and therefore one must measure the marginal product of medical care resources in units of health. Others would counter that health is too difficult to quantify, and that physician visits and hospital days are sufficient measures of output. By way of analogy, this group might point to studies of the automobile or wheat industries. Such studies typically look only at autos or bushels of wheat produced, and not at transportation services or nutrition. Similarly, one could consider the output of medical care to be the service purchased, and not take into account why the service was desired.

In this chapter we examine the issue of measuring the output of the medical care system. The discussion serves as important preliminary material for the analysis of planning and regulation in Chapter 6.

For some purposes a measure of output such as physician visits may be quite suitable. For example, if one wished to study the price of a visit (as was done in the earlier chapters), treating the visit as the product is by definition appropriate. Likewise, if one were describing physicians' productivity over a relatively short period of time, it may be sufficient to define their product as visits (over a long period of time, the assumption that the nature of the visit has not changed is untenable). Using the visit as a product, one can measure productivity by visits per physician-hour, just as one measures the productivity of automobile workers or farmers in terms of output per worker-hour. What reason, then, is there to concern ourselves with the relationship between medical care and health?

The reason for using more comprehensive dimensions of output than visits is the widespread public sector involvement in medical care. Public sector monies subsidize and public regulations control the production of medical care services. When public sector monies purchase goods or services, consumer preferences are typically not revealed in a market. Consequently, the public decisionmaker would like to know how consumers value the services bought with public funds.

Although the decisionmaker can never know the consumer's utility function, knowledge of the good's or service's ultimate effect is frequently useful in estimating the value consumers place on the good. For example, when comtemplating additional monies for the public schools, the School Board would like to know the effect of the additional resources on student learning, not simply what improvement will occur in teacher/student ratios or the square feet of space per student. Likewise, when contemplating changes in the national defense budget, the President is not so much interested in how the Army may change size, as in how that change affects the likelihood of war in various regions (an "output" even more difficult to measure than health). Analogously, because public monies purchase medical care services, one would like to measure those monies' effect on health.

The remainder of this chapter accepts the current public sector role in medical care and asks how to measure what public sector monies buy. In the next chapter I take up the question of the public sector's role. In effect, this chapter examines the relationship between medical care inputs and outputs; one might think of that relationship as a production function for health.

Early attempts to measure the output of the medical care system concentrated on the relationship between medical services and mortality, especially infant mortality, and between medical services and morbidity (sickness). Data in Table 5.1 describe time trends for mortality rates, along with the real increase in health expenditure. Column 1 shows actual (or crude) mortality rates (the ratio of deaths to the number of people alive at the time the Census is taken). These rates fell by a factor of almost two between 1900 and 1950, but since 1950 have been nearly constant. However, as a measure of changes in the likelihood of death, comparison of actual mortality rates over time is somewhat misleading. The population has been aging and more deaths occur in an elderly population. Therefore, even though death rates at each age may be the same, an older society will have a higher actual mortality rate than a younger society. For this reason, one should also compute age-adjusted mortality rates; such rates are shown in the second column of

Table 5.1 Mortality rates and expenditures

Year	Actual motality rate (per thousand)	Mortality rate age adjusted to 1940 population (per thousand)	Infant mortality (deaths per thousand live births)	Health expenditure‡ in billions of 1975 dollars (fiscal year)
1900	17.2*	17.8*	95.7†	n.a.
1920	13.0*	14.2*	76.7†	n.a.
1940	10.8	10.8	47.0	17.8
1950	9.6	8.4	29.2	37.8
1960	9.5	7.6	26.0	55.1
1965	9.4	7.4	24.7	73.3
1970	9.5	7.1	20.0	96.7
1975	9.0	6.4	16.1	122.2

Sources: Vital Statistics of the United States, 1972, Volume II, Part A, Tables 1-1, 1-2. *Statistical Abstract, 1976,* Tables 90 and 91. *Monthly Vital Statistics Report* 24:13. *Provisional Statistics, Annual Summary for the United States, 1975,* 30 June, 1976. *Forward Plan for Health, FY 78-82,* USDHEW, PHS, 1976. Robert M. Gibson and Marjorie S. Mueller, "National Health Expenditures, Fiscal Year 1976," *Social Security Bulletin* 40: Table 1 (April 1977), deflated by Medical Care component of Consumer Price Index .

*Ten states plus the District of Columbia.

†Based on data from birth registration states. 95.7 figure for 1915–1919; 76.7 figure for 1920–1924.

‡Most of these monies (87 percent in 1975) are for personal medical care services, but monies for medical research, government public health activities, and certain other expenditures are also included.

Table 5.1. These rates are an average of death rates at each age,[1] and they show a continuing fall. Likewise, there has been a steady fall in infant mortality, which is thought to be more sensitive to general medical conditions than is the overall mortality rate. The last column shows that concurrent with these declines in mortality rates, there has been a large rise in the amount of real medical services delivered.

---

1 Age adjustment presents an example of what economists call an index number problem. Age-adjusted mortality rates are computed by taking a weighted average of death rates at each age. The weights are usually taken to be the proportion of the population in each age group. However, the proportion in each age group will differ over time, so that the age-adjusted rates will depend on which year's population weights are chosen. (The 1940 population used in Table 5.1 is the population used in the United States Vital Statistics.) Moreover, the amount of change in the age-adjusted death rate will depend on which year's weights are chosen. If the year that was chosen has a relatively high proportion of the population in those age groups whose mortality rates fell, the age-adjusted rate will show more of a decrease and vice versa. However, it is not possible to say a priori whether age-adjusted rates will show a larger fall if earlier or later year population distributions are used.

This conclusion differs from the usual index number problem, computing

Data on morbidity have been collected only in more recent times. Table 5.2 shows data from the past twenty years on various types of disability days. The data appear to show no obvious pattern, but it is a mistake to rely on the untutored eye. In fact, there is no detectable trend over time in measures of restricted-activity days, bed-disability days, and school-loss days, but there is a statistically significant decline of about 0.5 days per ten years in the work-loss days measure. (This trend should not necessarily be extrapolated into the future.)

Overall one can conclude that over the twenty-five years from 1950 to 1975, age-adjusted mortality and one component of morbidity (workloss) have declined, while real expenditures on medical care services have grown slightly more than 4 percent per year. Real Gross National Product grew at a slower rate, only 3.3 percent over the same period, and the share of medical care in GNP grew from 4.5 percent in 1950 to 8.4 percent in 1975. Some rash souls might infer that the additional medical care services had purchased an increase in longevity. Such an inference, however, exemplifies a *post hoc, ergo propter hoc* fallacy; put another way, the observed association between health expenditure and health status change need not imply causation. As an illustration of how an association need not imply causation, consider cigarettes. The number of cigarettes consumed grew by more than 50 percent over the same twenty-five-year period (even per capita consumption rose), and few would claim that increasing cigarette consumption caused any improvement in mortality or morbidity rates.

What can be said about the role of medical care services in bringing about the improvement in mortality and morbidity? Several studies have examined how expenditure on medical care or access to medical care resources influence mortality and morbidity rates, *other factors held constant*. For the most part these studies have found little relationship between variation in medical resources and variation in measures of mortality and morbidity. For example, the authors of one study measured variation among states in age-adjusted mortality rates [1]. They adjusted statistically for state differ-

---

changes in real output. An index of real output sums the value of all products produced in a year, where value is measured by a given year's prices (analogous to a given year's population). Use of early-period prices will lead to a higher estimated growth rate than use of later-period prices. Because relative price and quantity of goods are negatively correlated, those items where quantity increases rapidly have a greater weight using early-period prices. For example, when television sets were first marketed in the 1940s, they had a relatively high price and relatively few were sold. Advances in technology caused their price to fall and the quantity sold to rise. If 1940s prices were used, television sets would get a relatively higher weight than if 1970s prices were used; because the consumption of television sets grew, the overall growth rate of output would be estimated to be higher using 1940s prices than using 1970s prices.

Table 5.2 Disability days per person per year

Year	Restricted-activity days*	Bed-disability days†	Work-loss days‡	School-loss days§
1957–1958	20.0	7.8	—	—
1958–1959	15.8	5.8	—	—
1959–1960	16.2	6.0	—	—
1961–1962	16.3	6.4	5.8	5.7
1963–1964	16.2	6.0	5.5	5.0
1965–1966	15.6	6.3	5.8	5.2
1968	15.3	6.3	5.4	4.9
1971	15.7	6.1	5.1	5.5
1972	16.7	6.5	5.3	5.3
1973	16.5	6.4	5.4	5.1
1974	17.2	6.7	4.9	5.6
1975	17.9	6.6	5.2	5.1

Sources: National Health Survey Publications, Series B, No. 29, Series 10, Nos. 4, 24, 90, 100, 115.

*A restricted-activity day is one on which a person cuts down on his or her usual activities for the whole of that day because of illness or injury.

†A bed-disability day is one on which a person stays in bed for all or most of the day because of illness or injury.

‡A work-loss day is one on which a person age seventeen and over did not work at a job or business for at least half the normal workday because of illness or injury. The denominator is currently employed persons.

§A school-loss day is one on which a person age six to sixteen did not attend school because of illness or injury.

ences in income, education, degree of urbanization, percentage employed in manufacturing, consumption of alcohol and cigarettes per capita, and presence of a medical school. Holding these factors constant, the authors estimated that states that spent 10 percent more on medical care might reduce their mortality rate by 1 percent. However, the 1 percent figure is not estimated with much precision, and in fact the true figure could well be zero (i.e., no reduction from increased expenditure). The results of this study typify studies of the relationship between medical care resources and the overall mortality rate.

A modification of this approach is to examine the relationship between medical care resources and the infant mortality rate. Although limiting the study to infant mortality will give only a partial picture of the productivity of medical resources, infant mortality is thought to provide a favorable opportunity to observe a relationship between medical care resources and health outcomes. Perhaps the most comprehensive examination of infant mortality and medical resources was conducted using a sample of 134,000 live births in New York City in 1968 [2]. The authors adjusted for several factors known or thought to be associated with infant mortality, including the education of the mother, her age, her ethnic group, her marital status, and how many children she already had. In addition, the authors adjusted for certain medical conditions associated with infant mortality, such as the presence of diabetes or an inadequate pelvis. After making these adjustments, the authors examined how infant mortality related to the "adequacy" of medical care services. Adequacy was defined as having a visit in the first three months of pregnancy, having nine or more prenatal visits if the gestation period was nine months or longer, and having a personal physician (rather than an intern or resident) admit and care for the mother at the time of delivery. Using this definition of adequacy, the authors showed that if babies of mothers with less than adequate care had the same death rate as babies of mothers with adequate care, the infant mortality rate would have fallen from 21.8 per 1,000 live births to 18.4 per thousand, a reduction of 16 percent [2, Table 1-13].

One could criticize the study's definition of adequacy as arbitrary, but that is quibbling. Unfortunately, there is a more fundamental problem. The study compares infant mortality among babies of mothers who sought care early and regularly during their pregnancy with babies of mothers who did not. Although the authors made a number of adjustments to achieve comparability between the two groups of mothers, it is unlikely that the remaining difference in outcomes between these two groups was solely attributable to medical care. More precisely, if medical care had been extended to those mothers who did not obtain it, it is unlikely that the outcome would be the same as among those mothers who did receive the adequate care. Mothers who sought medical care early and regularly in their pregnancy were undoubtedly more motivated to pay attention to diet, weight, exercise, and other factors under the mother's control that affect infant mortality. Such unmeasured factors could possibly explain the *entire* difference between the two groups, although this seems unlikely. Nonetheless, the 16 percent difference is almost certainly not attributable solely to medical care. Thus we are left with an uncertain estimate of the relationship between medical care and infant mortality.

Review of the literature reveals little evidence that *further* investments in medical care services will lead to any marked reductions in overall mortality and morbidity rates.[2] Examining causes of death reinforces such a conclusion. Table 5.3 shows the seven leading causes of death in three age groups. Over half of all deaths among children ages five to fourteen are accounted for by accidents, and the next leading cause of death is malignant

---

2 A similar conclusion is reached by Victor Fuchs [3, Chapter 2], whose writings have significantly contributed to this chapter's analysis. See also [4].

Table 5.3 Seven leading causes of death, 1972, in three age groups

Cause	Death rate (per hundred thousand)
Age 5–14	
All causes	40.8
Motor vehicle accidents	10.7
Accidents other than motor vehicle	10.0
Malignant neoplasms	5.5
Congenital anomalies	2.4
Major cardiovascular diseases	1.7
Influenza and pneumonia	1.4
Homicide	0.9
Age 35–44	
All causes	302.1
Major cardiovascular diseases	81.2
Malignant neoplasms	57.7
Motor vehicle accidents	24.2
Accidents other than motor vehicle	20.9
Cirrhosis of liver	20.3
Suicide	16.8
Homicide	16.2
Age 65–74	
All causes	3,256.9
Major cardiovascular diseases	1,986.9
Malignant neoplasms	774.1
Diabetes mellitus	89.7
Influenza and pneumonia	86.7
Accidents other than motor vehicle	48.9
Cirrhosis of liver	43.1
Motor vehicle accidents	32.1

Source: Vital Statistics of the United States, 1972.

neoplasms (cancer). Mortality from accidents might be decreased somewhat by improved emergency services, but it seems unlikely that additional medical care services for this age group would have any effect on its mortality rate. By the time of middle age (thirty-five to forty-four), cardiovascular (heart) disease and cancer are the leading causes of death, accounting for nearly half the deaths. Improved emergency services and greater control of high blood pressure have probably played a role in reducing the toll from heart disease over the past fifteen years, but it is problematical whether further extension of medical care services can reduce mortality from any of these causes substantially. A similar conclusion holds in the age group from sixty-five to seventy-four, where over three-fourths of deaths are accounted for by cardiovascular disease and malignant neoplasms.

What then accounts for the widespread impression of a relationship between medical services and health? Some may confuse total (or average) effect with marginal effect. Eliminating medical care services altogether could lead to a marked increase in mortality and morbidity rates, even though a further increase in medical services would show little effect.

Others may confuse the effect of more services given existing technology with more services given an improved technology. (I am using technology to mean knowledge of disease processes and techniques for intervention, not just machines.) Technology has radically changed in this century, giving the physician weapons that did not previously exist. Examining the leading causes of death over time (Table 5.4) shows the impact of technological change. The first five causes of death listed in the table represent categories that were important in 1900 and to some degree in 1940, but are virtually nonexistent in 1970. (By contrast, heart disease, cancer, and motor vehicle accidents have all increased in importance.) The decline in the first five categories of death can be partially ascribed to the discovery of antibiotics and vaccines (as well as improved sanitation and nutrition), and so the physician's ability to affect health (the productivity of physician time) has improved. Even though additional medical care services may be productive as technology changes, it does not follow that additional services with a given technology will be very productive. Figure 5.1 illustrates this point. Using

Table 5.4 Causes of death in various years—death rates per hundred thousand

Cause of death	1900*	1940	1970
Total	1,719.1	1,076.5	945.3
Tuberculosis, all forms	194.4	45.9	2.6
Gastritis, duodenitis, enteritis, colitis	142.7	10.3	0.6
Influenza and pneumonia	202.2	70.3	30.9
Diphtheria	40.3	1.1	0.05
Typhoid and paratyphoid fever	31.3	1.1	0.05
Major cardiovascular renal diseases	345.2	485.7	496.0
Malignant neoplasms	64.0	120.3	162.8
Motor vehicle accidents	0.4†	26.2	26.9
Accidents other than motor vehicles	72.3	29.8	21.2

*Based on data from ten death registration states plus the District of Columbia.

†Figure for 1906 (earliest figure available).

Source: Bureau of the Census, Historical Statistics of the United States, Colonial Times to 1970, Part I, p. 58. Washington. D.C.: Government Printing Office, 1975.

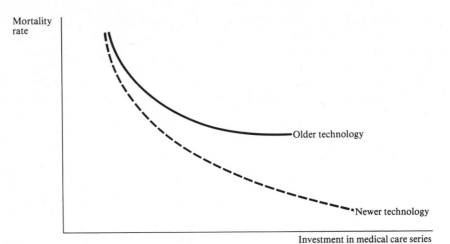

Mortality rate

Older technology

Newer technology

Investment in medical care series

Fig. 5.1 Hypothesized relationships between investment in medical care resources and mortality rates. Newer technology may make medical care resources considerably more productive.

the older technology, one encounters diminishing returns much more rapidly than using the newer technology.

Because of technological change's importance in generating improvements in health, the United States has invested heavily in biomedical research. Approximately $5 billion were devoted to such research in 1975, with $2 billion of that coming from the National Institutes of Health (see Table 3.3). The quantitative relationship between research expenditure and the mortality rate cannot be precisely established, although undoubtedly they are linked.

The data on cause of death (Table 5.3) make clear the importance to mortality of an individual's life-style. Diet, obesity, and cigarette smoking have all been linked with cardiovascular disease; cigarettes and environmental pollutants have been linked to cancer; excessive alcohol consumption causes cirrhosis of the liver; and driving fast without wearing a seat belt increases the death rate from motor vehicle accidents.

Therefore, identification of the current leading causes of death and comparison with the leading causes of 1900 lead one to the inference that life-style and improved medical technology have more to do with mortality than additional resources in medical care. This conclusion is supported by examination of data from the United States National Health Survey on certain physiological measures of an individual's health [5]. These measures included blood pressure, cholesterol levels, abnormal electrocardiograms, abnormal chest X-rays, and the state of one's gums. Unfortunately, the most recent data on adults come from the early 1960s. At that time age and sex explained individual variation in these measures but the quantity of medical care resources in the individual's place of residence did not.[3] In other words, if those areas with fewer resources were to obtain additional resources, one would predict little change in these physiological measures; conversely, if the well-endowed areas had somewhat fewer resources, one would also predict little change in these measures.

By contrast the better educated have better gums and a lower prevalence of abnormal chest X-rays (holding income constant). The better educated may also have a lower prevalence of high blood pressure. Income also affects these measures. Holding education constant, higher-income individuals have healthier gums and a lower prevalence of abnormal chest X-rays. Income and education probably influence these measures of health through their effect on live-style. Exactly which differences in life-style are important to health is uncertain, but diet, housing, and exercise are likely candidates.

In sum, these results support the hypothesis that life-style affects health status more than the medical care resources in an area. Because increased medical resources affect health through increased consumption of medical care services (see Chapter 4), one infers that life-style is more important than increased consumption of services.

Few have explored the relationship between medical care services and morbidity. One study examined days of work lost because of illness or injury in twenty-two metropolitan areas [6]. Among younger workers (ages seventeen to forty-four), additional physician visits were associated with *more* work loss; there was no association among workers ages forty-five to sixty-four. This result, which may seem puzzling at first, could occur if the physician advised the sick patient to go home and go to bed, whereas the individual who never consulted the physician might continue to work. Of course, the individual who does not consult the physician may thereby prolong the illness. Nonetheless, the odds appear to be in one's favor if one is young, whereas the odds appear approximately even when one is over forty-five (given the failure of a relationship between physician visits and work loss to appear in the older age group).

Some life-style variables are important in explaining work-loss days; work loss is higher among older workers in cities with high concentrations of poverty; work loss is higher among younger workers in cities with low per capita food expenditures, and with high proportions of the population completing high school. This latter result could be caused by more extensive sick-leave provisions among individuals who have completed high school (assuming that more extensive sick leave causes a worker to take a day off

---

3 Drugs that lowered abnormally high blood pressures became widely used after these data were collected; thus, there might now be a relationship between the quantity of medical resources and the number of persons with high blood pressure. When more recent data become available, this hypothesis can be tested.

more readily). Thus these results are also consistent with the hypothesis that at the margin medical care does not affect morbidity as much as life-style.

What, then, does the marginal unit of medical care buy? If it does not cause notable improvements in mortality and morbidity, why do individuals not reduce their consumption of medical care? One answer can be found in extensive insurance; fully insured people should use medical care until its marginal product is approximately zero. Hospital services provide the best test of such a prediction, for even in 1964–1965 they were over 80 percent insured. Data collected at that time suggest that a substantial fraction of the hospital's resources went to individuals in their last year of life. More specifically, over 20 percent of hospital expenditures on individuals over twenty-five were made on behalf of individuals in their last year of life.[4] The percentage has surely risen since that time; a reasonable guess would be that it is now 25 to 30 percent, perhaps more.[5] Undoubtedly some of these resources have little chance of benefiting the terminally ill patient; if so, the resources have a near zero marginal product. Thus, extensive insurance may induce use of resources until their marginal product is near zero.

Outpatient services, however, are not so well insured, and the user pays an opportunity cost in time. (The hospitalized patient may be sufficiently sick that the opportunity cost of time spent in the hospital is negligible.) Yet the average person makes just under four visits to the physician's office each year. Such visits would be predicted to have a positive marginal product for the same reason that hospital services would be predicted to have a near zero marginal product. But what is the marginal product of the office visit? What motivates the consumer to pay time and money costs if the return at the margin in terms of mortality or morbidity is low?

---

4 This figure is computed on the basis of data in National Center for Health Statistics [7], which show the number of decedents and median expenditure among the decedents and nondecedents. I have assumed that the ratio of the medians equals the ratio of the means. (There are no data, but this assumption is unlikely to be far wrong.) National Center for Health Statistics [8] contain data on the total number of hospitalized individuals in the over-twenty-five population.

5 Three factors will have caused the figure to rise: (1) the Medicare Program was implemented immediately after these data were collected. Data show that only 42 percent of decedents sixty-five and over had hospital insurance in the pre-Medicare period [9]. Because of the Medicare program, this figure is now nearly 100 percent. (2) Technological change has made dying more costly. Intensive care units were few in 1963 and 1964, whereas now the sickest patients are generally in intensive care units and a high proportion of deaths in the hospital probably take place there. (I have found no data.) Intensive care units are much more expensive to operate than routine wards. (3) A declining birth rate has meant fewer hospital resources are devoted to normal deliveries, the leading cause of hospitalization. Between 1964 and 1975, the fraction of hospital discharges accounted for by normal deliveries fell from 15 to 9 percent (computed from [10, 11]).

The predominant output of many outpatient visits may be relief of anxiety, relief of pain, and provision of prognostic information. The difficulty of measuring such outputs does not make them less real. Some individuals will be told their chest pain is a muscle spasm and not a heart problem. Others will have their athlete's foot cured. Visits for such problems will certainly not change the mortality statistics and are unlikely to change the disability day statistics. Yet the individuals treated will probably assess the time and money to visit the physician as well spent.

The hypothesis that the marginal unit of medical care has little to do with mortality and morbidity receives inferential support from the relationship between a country's income and its expenditure on medical care. Of interest is whether expenditure on medical care rises more than proportionately with income (whether the income elasticity exceeds one). Economists call goods with such a characteristic luxuries—fine wines and foreign travel are two examples. By contrast, when spending rises less than proportionately with income (income elasticity is less than one), the good is termed a necessity—food is an example. Relatively cheap medical interventions that could alter mortality and morbidity would almost surely be necessities; most everyone would want them. On the other hand, heroic measures near the end of life, symptomatic relief, and reductions in anxiety might well be luxuries, goods whose consumption rises more than proportionately with the income of a society.

Figure 5.2 shows a line that has been fit to the level of medical care spending and the Gross Domestic Product (GDP) per capita of thirteen countries.[6] As can be seen, the expenditure of most countries falls quite close to the line, so GDP predicts medical expenditure well; in fact, variation in income across countries explains 92 percent of the variation in medical care expenditure. The equation of the line is:

Medical expenditure $= -60 + .0788$ (GDP per capita).

Dividing both sides of the equation by GDP per capita shows that the share of Gross Domestic Product spent on medical care *rises* with income, as depicted in Fig. 5.3.[7] This shows that the estimated income elasticity exceeds one. A similar pattern has been found over time within a wide variety of

6 Gross Domestic Product has very minor definitional differences from Gross National Product, but for practical purposes is the same.
7 This estimated equation in Fig. 5.3 is Share $= 8.16 - 6883/$GDP. The t-statistic on the 6883 figure is 4.00, significant at 1 percent. A similar result is found by Kleiman [12], whose sample includes both developed and less-developed countries. If all variables in his equation predicting health expenditure are set at their average sample value, the estimated income elasticity is 1.22, and the estimated elasticity remains above one as income varies.

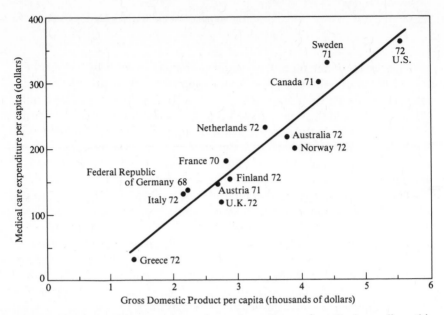

Fig. 5.2 Relationship between gross domestic product and medical spending, thirteen countries. The numbers following the names of the countries are the last two digits of the year of observation. (*Source*: Newhouse, Joseph P., "Income and Medical Care Expenditure Across Countries," P-5608-1, The Rand Corporation, Santa Monica, California, August 1976, p. 4.)

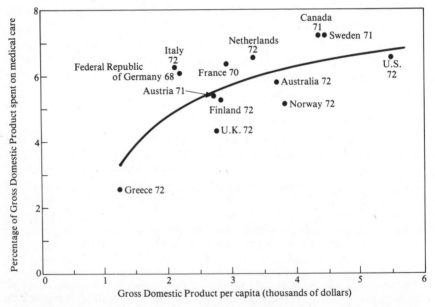

Fig. 5.3 Relationship between gross domestic product and share spent on medical care in thirteen countries (recent years). (*Source*: Newhouse, Joseph P., "Income and Medical Care Expenditure Across Countries," P-5608-1, The Rand Corporation, Santa Monica, California, August 1976, p. 7.)

countries. As countries have grown wealthier, they have spent a larger fraction of their Gross Domestic Product on medical care.

Thus, data from different countries at (approximately) one point in time, as well as data from within countries over time, indicate that the income elasticity of medical care exceeds one (in the range of current medical care expenditure). Such a finding supports the inference that the marginal unit of medical care is not a simple intervention to alter mortality and morbidity. Rather, the marginal unit appears to produce subjective services that may well be desired, but are extraordinarily difficult to measure. Assuming this is the case, how do we know what the marginal product of medical care resources is, or how much medical care is wanted? The final chapter addresses these issues.

REFERENCES

1. Richard Auster, Irving Leveson, and Deborah Sarachek. "The Production of Health: An Exploratory Study." *Journal of Human Resources* 4, No. 4: 411–436 (Fall 1969).

2. D. M. Kessner et al. *Infant Death: An Analysis of Maternal Risk and Health Care.* Washington, D.C.: Institute of Medicine, National Academy of Sciences, 1973.

3. Victor Fuchs. *Who Shall Live?* New York: Basic Books, 1974.

4. Lee and Alexandra Benham, "The Impact of Incremental Medical Services on Health Status, 1963–1970." In *Equity in Health Services,* edited by Ronald Andersen, Joanna Kravitz, and Odin Anderson. Cambridge: Ballinger, 1975.

5. Joseph P. Newhouse and Lindy J. Friedlander. "The Relationship Between Medical Resources and Measures of Health: Some Additional Evidence." Santa Monica: The Rand Corporation, R-2066-HEW, 1977.

6. Joseph P. Newhouse. "Determinants of Days Lost from Work Due to Sickness." Reprint from *Empirical Studies in Health Economics,* edited by Herbert Klarman. Baltimore, Md.: Johns Hopkins Press, 1970.

7. National Center for Health Statistics. "Expenses for Hospital and Institutional Care During the Last Year of Life for Adults Who Died in 1964 or 1965, United States." Washington, D.C.: Government Printing Office, 1971 (Data from the National Health Survey: Series 22, No. 11).

8. National Center for Health Statistics. "Current Estimates from the Health Interview Survey, United States—July 1964–June 1965." Washington, D.C.: Government Printing Office, 1965 (Data from the National Health Survey: Series 10, No. 25).

9. National Health Center for Health Statistics. "Health Insurance Coverage of Adults Who Died in 1964 or 1965, United States." Washington, D.C.: Government Printing Office, 1969 (Data from the National Health Survey: Series 22, No. 10).

10. National Center for Health Statistics. "Patients Discharged from Short-Stay Hospitals, United States: October–December 1964." Washington, D.C.: Government Printing Office, 1966 (Data from the National Health Survey: Series 13, No. 1).

11. National Center for Health Statistics. "Utilization of Short-Stay Hospitals: Annual Summary for the United States, 1975." Washington, D.C.: Government Printing Office, 1977 (Data from the National Health Survey: Series 13, No. 31).

12. Ephraim Kleiman. "Determinants of National Outlay on Health." In *The Economics of Health and Medical Care: Proceedings of a Conference Held by the International Economic Association at Tokyo,* edited by Mark Perlman. London: Macmillan, 1974.

Plan and Market 6 Alternatives to the Status Quo: Techniques for Managing Resource Allocation in Medical Care

All societies must answer certain questions when organizing the production of medical care services and other goods. How much medical care will be produced? With what techniques will medical care services be produced? Who will receive medical care services? How much will providers of medical care services be paid? Answers to these questions are importantly influenced by the market structure of medical care, that is, the reliance placed upon competitive market forces relative to the role given public utility regulation or health planning. This chapter explores the choice between competitive and regulated market structures.

THE PROPERTIES OF PERFECTLY COMPETITIVE MARKETS

As background for the discussion, we review in the next few pages how the preceding questions are answered in an economy with perfectly competitive markets. We shall look not only at how, but also at how well a competitive market answers these questions. The current market for medical care is not perfectly competitive (see Chapter 4), of course, but an understanding of competitive markets is necessary to appraise both the current organization of the medical care market and proposed alternatives to it. In order to employ graphical techniques, we will limit attention to a two-good, two-factor, two-person economy. The reader will have to take on faith that the results generalize to a many-good, many-factor, many-person economy. For convenience, let us call the two factors of production in the economy labor and capital, and let us call the two goods medical care and COMP (the subsequent discussion summarizes an article by Bator [1] to which the reader is referred for further details.)

Perfect competition (with certain additional assumptions) achieves a criterion known as *Pareto optimality*. (Pareto optimality is sometimes called efficiency.) If the outcome is Pareto optimal, no person can be made better off without making someone else worse off. Conversely, unless an outcome is Pareto optimal, all persons can be made better off. This desirable property makes Pareto optimality a standard for judging alternative arrangements for organizing production.

We now show why perfect competition is Pareto optimal. We begin by supposing that a certain amount of labor and capital is available to produce goods and services. Figure 6.1 illustrates the amount of labor and capital available. The distance between points A and B represents the amount of labor available, and the distance between points A and C the amount of capital available.[1] One can draw in isoquants for the production of medical care from the labor and capital. Two such isoquants are shown in Fig. 6.1 and are labeled 1 and 2. There are an infinite number of others that are not drawn but have the same general shape. The points along isoquant 1 show various combinations of labor and capital that will produce a constant amount of medical care. So do the points along isoquant 2; however, the amount of medical care produced by the combinations of labor and capital represented by isoquant 2 is greater than the combinations represented by isoquant 1. Looked at another way, isoquant 2 represents devoting to medical care a greater share of the labor and capital available for all uses.

Now turn the book upside down. The isoquants labeled 3 and 4 are for COMP. At point D, no labor or capital is devoted to producing COMP; it is all producing medical care. (Where is the point at which no medical care is produced?) Let us suppose this society is currently dividing its labor and capital between medical care and COMP in a manner represented by point P. An amount of medical care corresponding to isoquant 1 is being produced, and an amount of COMP corresponding to isoquant 4 is being produced. This society is *not* at a Pareto optimal point, because any move from P into the shaded area will increase the production of both medical care and COMP. More medical care will be produced because the new medical care isoquant lies northeast of isoquant 1 (toward isoquant 2), and more of COMP will be produced because the new isoquant for COMP will lie southwest of isoquant 4. (Recall that no production of COMP occurs at point D and southwesterly moves from D represent increased production of COMP; for example, isoquant 4 represents more of COMP than isoquant 3.) If more of both goods can be produced, everyone can be made better off (a little bit more can be given to everybody); hence, point P cannot be a Pareto optimal point.

---

1 This entire diagram is called an Edgeworth-Bowley box diagram.

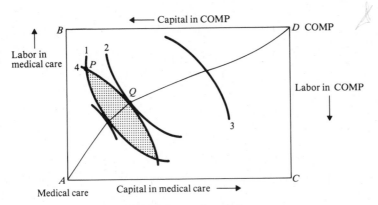

Fig. 6.1 Production possibilities for labor and capital.

Point P cannot be a Pareto optimal point because the slopes of the iso-quants for the two goods at point P are not equal. At point P medical care uses a considerable amount of labor and relatively little capital, while the opposite is true for COMP. For example, one might be able to keep production of medical care at a constant level by giving up three units of labor and receiving one more unit of capital. However, one might also be able to keep the production of COMP constant by giving up three units of capital and receiving one more unit of labor. (Draw in such changes along the isoquant.) Suppose producers of medical care give up one unit of labor to producers of COMP and receive in exchange one unit of capital. Because production of medical care can be kept constant by giving up three units of labor if one more unit of capital is received, there are two units of labor "left over" to produce more medical care than had been produced on isoquant 1. (Trace through what happens to the production of COMP when more labor is received.) Thus, reallocation of factors between the two goods can increase the production of both. A reallocation of this kind can always take place unless the slopes of the isoquants are equal; equality occurs where the isoquants are tangent to each other and is a necessary condition for efficiency in production.

The locus of points where the isoquants are tangent is represented by the upward-sloping line that begins at point A and terminates at point D; this line is called a contract curve. From the contract curve one can derive the production-possibility curve for this society shown in Fig. 6.2. The production-possibility curve, which shows the maximum amount of medical care that can be produced for any given amount of COMP, is derived simply by reading off the levels of production of the two goods that are represented by the isoquants as they cut across the contract curve. Thus, the points A and D are the extreme points of the production-possibility curve; point Q in Fig.

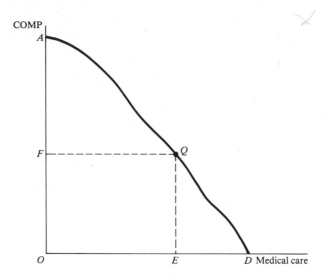

Fig. 6.2 Society's production possibility curve.

6.1 represents an amount of medical care equal to that represented by iso-quant 2 and an amount of COMP represented by isoquant 4, and is shown as point Q in Fig. 6.2 also.

Perfect competition assures that society is producing on the production-possibility curve and not somewhere within it. Why? (See if you can answer before reading on.) If perfect competition prevails, firms will be minimizing the cost of production, and they will produce where the slope of the iso-quant equals the price ratio of the two factors (see Chapter 3). But because each firm uses the same two factors and faces the same price ratio for those factors, the slope of the isoquant at the point each firm produces is the same. Thus, the isoquants of different firms will be tangent, and so perfectly competitive firms will be on the contract curve. Put another way, for point P, which is off the contract curve, to be a least-cost point for firms producing medical care and also for firms producing COMP, the firms would have to face different price ratios for labor and capital. But this is not possible in a competitive market.

Suppose, then, that firms produce on the contract curve and that the so-ciety is on its production-possibility curve. Suppose that a certain amount of medical care and COMP are being produced, as shown by point Q. Fig. 6.2 shows two dotted lines that form a box within the production-possibility curve, somewhat like the box in Fig. 6.1. Figure 6.3 shows the box in dashed lines from Fig. 6.2. Point Q defines an amount of medical care (OE in Fig. 6.2) and an amount of COMP (OF in Fig. 6.2) being produced by the firms in our perfectly competitive economy. This amount of medical care is repre-sented by the horizontal line in Fig. 6.3, and the amount of COMP is repre-

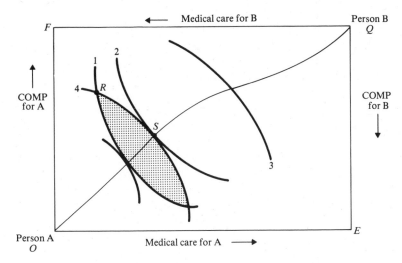

Fig. 6.3 Consumption possibilities.

sented by the vertical line in Fig. 6.3. Inside the box in Fig. 6.3 are indifference curves (instead of isoquants as in Fig. 6.1). The indifference curve labeled 1 belongs to person A, and shows the combinations of medical care and COMP that would leave person A equally well off. (If you are hazy about the notion of indifference curves, refer back to Chapter 2.) Indifference curve 2 also belongs to A, and points on indifference curve 2 are preferred to indifference curve 1. Indifference curves 3 and 4 belong to person B (turn the page upside down if this is not clear). Suppose the amount of medical care and COMP that each person receives is shown by point R. Then both individuals can be made better off by a move into the shaded area. It is the same story as in Fig. 6.1; person A values medical care (relative to COMP) more highly than person B when both persons are at point R. Hence both are better off if person B trades person A some medical care and receives COMP in exchange. Mutually beneficial trades are possible so long as the two persons place different (relative) valuations on the two goods. They place the same (relative) valuation on the goods when the indifference curves are tangent. (Suppose each would give up one unit of COMP for two units of medical care; then no mutually beneficial trade is possible.) The line running from southwest to northeast shows the locus of points at which the indifference curves are tangent and is another contract curve. It defines the points at which mutually beneficial trades are not possible (known as efficiency in exchange).

Perfect competition ensures that society operates on this contract curve also. Why? If both persons maximize their utility, each will purchase a combination of goods where the slope of the indifference curve equals the ratio of the prices of the two goods (Fig. 2.1). With perfect competition both consumers face the same (market) price for the two goods, so the slopes of their indifference curves will be equal at the utility-maximizing point, exactly the condition required for being on the contract curve.

One additional condition is needed for Pareto optimality. Suppose at point S in Fig. 6.3 the slope of both indifference curves does not equal the slope of the production possibility curve at point Q in Fig. 6.2. The slope at Q defines the real (production) possibilities for giving up one good to obtain more of another. For example, suppose the slope at Q is -1, so that two more units of COMP can be obtained if two units of medical care are given up. However, suppose the slopes of the indifference curves at S show that each consumer would feel equally well off by giving up one unit of COMP for two units of medical care. In that case, the two persons should each give up two units of medical care. They will get two units of COMP (as per the production-possibility curve), but they are now better off, because they would have been equally well off with one more unit of COMP (as per the indifference curve). For this kind of reallocation not to be beneficial to both parties, the slope of the indifference curve must equal the slope of the pro- duction-possibility curve.

Again this condition is satisfied in perfect competition. The real rate of transformation between the two goods (the slope at Q) must equal the price ratio of the two goods. If this condition does not hold, it will pay someone to produce less of one good and more of the other. For example, suppose medical care and COMP both sell for $10 per unit, but if one unit of medical care is given up, two units of COMP can be produced. Firms producing medical care will find the production of COMP more profitable, and will shift out of medical care until the price ratio between the two goods equals the real rate of transformation. Because utility-maximizing con- sumers purchase so as to leave the slope of their indifference curves equal to the price ratio, the slope of the indifference curves will equal the slope of the production-possibility frontier in perfect competition.

Suppose now that S in Fig. 6.3 represents a point at which the slope of the indifference curve equals the slope of the production-possibility curve. (There may be more than one such point on the contract curve in Fig. 6.3.) Such points are points on an indifference curve for each person (for example, point S is a point on indifference curves 2 and 4). Thus, point S represents a distribution of utility between the two persons. Figure 6.4 shows the distribution of utility represented by all points that have the same properties as point S (on the contract curve and the slope of the indifference curve equals the slope of the production-possibility curve; one or more such points correspond to each point on the production-possibility curve). The downward-sloping line in this figure is called the utility-possibility frontier. (more precisely, the frontier is the locus of the outermost points of all points that have the properties of point S.) The frontier shows the maximum possible utility for each person, holding the other person's utility constant.

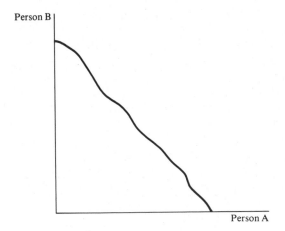

Fig. 6.4 Utility possibility frontier.

To operate inside the utility-possibility frontier is to be in a position where all persons can be made better off, and is therefore not a Pareto optimal outcome.

By definition, all points on the line in Fig. 6.4 are Pareto optimal. From any point on the line one person can be made better off only if the other is made worse off. Perfect competition is compatible with all points on the line. The initial distribution of income between the two persons will determine which point on this curve is the actual outcome. (Recall that in Fig. 6.3 a consumer's income or budget constraint determines how high an indifference curve the person can reach.)

We have demonstrated a basic postulate of welfare economics. Perfect competition brings about an optimal outcome in the following sense: No one can be made better off without making someone else worse off. To argue that someone should be made better off at the expense of someone else (e.g., the rich should be taxed and the proceeds used to benefit the poor) is to argue that the income distribution is not acceptable. This result—that perfect competition achieves Pareto optimality—is an important argument for relying on market forces in medical care. What are arguments against relying on market forces?

PROBLEMS CONNECTED WITH ORGANIZING THE MEDICAL CARE SECTOR TO RESEMBLE A PERFECTLY COMPETITIVE MARKET

Equity considerations lead to the first criticism of market organization. Some argue that the consumption of medical care services should not depend on ability to pay (income); a less extreme position is that medical care consumption should not be overly dependent on ability to pay. Put more technically, medical care should exhibit a near-zero income elasticity of demand, holding the health status of the individual constant. Charging market prices for medical care does not lead to a near-zero income elasticity of demand. Hence most agree that the outcome of an unadulterated price system is not acceptable, at least for the poor.

For many years the price system has been modified by charging the poor person less for medical services; economists refer to such seemingly well-intentioned arrangements as price discrimination. It may surprise you, but price discrimination is not consistent with Pareto optimality. To see why not, refer back to Fig. 6.3. Suppose person A is poor and person B is wealthy. If they are charged different (relative) prices for medical care and COMP, they will be at a point such as R, off the contract curve. (Each will move to the point where the budget line is tangent to the indifference curve, but with different price ratios the indifference curves will not be tangent at that point.) The inconsistency between price discrimination and Pareto optimality may be counterintuitive. If so, it may help to work through an example to see how problems arise.

Suppose oranges are 25 cents a pound for wealthy people, but only 10 cents a pound for poor people. Candy bars, however, are 20 cents for everybody. If an individual maximizes utility subject to a budget constraint, the marginal utility of the last unit of a good purchased divided by its price is equal for all goods. (If these ratios are not equal, show that the individual is not maximizing utility.) Equivalently, the last pound of oranges bought by the wealthy person yields that person 25 cents worth of utility, while the last candy bar bought yields 20 cents worth of utility. The poor person, however, values the last pound of oranges purchased at 10 cents, and the last candy bar at 20 cents. It is worthwhile for the poor person to trade the wealthy person oranges for candy bars. Suppose the poor person trades the wealthy person a pound of oranges for a candy bar. The poor person has given up something valued at 10 cents and received something valued at 20 cents; the wealthy person has given up something that the wealthy person values at 20 cents, but received something valued at 25 cents. Thus, both are better off, and if both can be made better off, they were not at a Pareto optimal point.

Barter need not have been employed. The poor person could have sold the wealthy person a pound of oranges for 20 cents. The wealthy person would be better off buying oranges for 20 cents a pound rather than 25 cents; the poor person would make a profit of 10 cents per pound. If such sales are not to occur when price discrimination exists, the good must be nontransferable between persons; I can resell oranges to you, but I cannot resell you my physician visit. Hence, price discrimination is not possible for oranges, but is possible for physician visits.

Price discrimination is per se evidence of monopoly power. Suppose oranges cost 15 cents a pound to grow, and selling them to wealthy individuals at the price of 25 cents a pound generates enough profits to cover the loss incurred when they are sold to poor individuals at a price of 10 cents a pound. In that case, there will be a profitable opportunity for entry by another firm to sell oranges to wealthy persons for a price between 15 and 25 cents. As such entry occurs, the price to the wealthy person will be forced down toward 15 cents and price to the poor person will be forced up toward 15 cents (because costs must be covered by the orange grower).

Is elimination of price discrimination an example of the compassionless operation of the market that has been portrayed by novelists and social reformers for at least two centuries? Is it a basis for condemning market organization? Recall the basic postulate of welfare economics. Perfect competition is Pareto optimal. If the distribution of income is acceptable, one cannot do better than the perfectly competitive result. If the distribution of income is *not* acceptable, it may be preferable to sell medical services to poor persons at a lower price. But economic analysis alerts us to two implications: (1) Such an outcome is possible only if the good is not transferable and if entry to the industry is controlled; otherwise, new firms will enter the wealthy person market. (2) Even more importantly, a still better outcome could be achieved by transferring cash income between the wealthy person and the poor person (p. 93). In fact, it is possible for the wealthy person to pay the poor person some money and leave them both better off, provided the price discrimination ends. This represents a move from point R in Fig 6.3 into the shaded area.

Thus equity arguments against market organization in medical care can be answered by appropriate redistribution of income. Whether the redistribution will take place is uncertain, but equity considerations should pose no absolute bar to market organization. Moreover, price discrimination is not Pareto optimal.

At this point, however, a second criticism of market organization may be raised. We have just shown that if price discrimination ends, both poor and wealthy individuals can be made better off *as they view their utility*. But is their view appropriate? In Chapter 4 we discussed consumers' ignorance about the benefit of medical care services. Even if we exclude a malevolent physician's manipulating the patient for the physician's gain, a well-intentioned physician does not know with certainty the consumer's utility function. As a result, if the consumer knew as much about the technical possibilities as the physician does (i.e., knows as well as the physician does how much medical care services can be of benefit), the consumer might choose to consume more or fewer medical services than the physician recommends.[2]

Suppose the tastes of the well-informed consumer are the standard used to judge resource allocation. If the actual outcome with market organization diverges markedly from the outcome if consumers were perfectly informed, market organization may not be optimal. Further, the consumer may be aware of ignorance and choose to delegate choice to a regulator. The extent of consumer ignorance is a central issue in the debate over the organization of medical services, and we shall return to it below.

Another objection to market organization, in addition to equity and consumer ignorance, is the assumption that markets are everywhere perfectly competitive. If all markets are not perfectly competitive, it does not necessarily improve matters to institute competition in a single market. Hence, because all other markets are not perfectly competitive, perfect competition in medical care might not be optimal.[3] In practice, such an objection to competition in a particular sector does not carry much force. The burden of proof is usually placed on those arguing against competition in a single market; they must show why society would be worse off. No one is seriously arguing against competition in medical care for this reason, and I believe this general theoretical objection has little practical relevance to the present discussion.

A final objection to a perfectly competitive market in medical care is the risk it places on individuals. Because the incidence of illness is uncertain, most individuals desire insurance to protect them against random losses (see Chapter 2), and an optimal arrangement would almost surely include such protection. Insurance as presently written usually reimburses a certain proportion (frequently all) of medical care bills and so provides protection against random losses, but the premium paid for such insurance does not reflect an individual's expenditure on medical care. By protecting the individual in this fashion, insurance causes two departures from the competitive model. First, insurance subsidizes the marginal unit of medical care. The

---

2 Sometimes the argument is made that the price system is pernicious because it discourages the consumption of efficacious preventive care, thereby raising long-run expenditure. In effect, the argument is that consumers do not purchase a good that is in their long-run best interests. Two responses might be made to this argument. First, few preventive medical care services have been demonstrated to be efficacious (immunizations are an exception). Second, if it can be shown that the price system deters consumption of efficacious preventive services, they can be subsidized or even made available free of charge. A related argument is that prices deter individuals with treatable illnesses who have symptoms from seeking medical care at a time when medical care can cheaply alter the course of the disease. The experiment described in Chapter 2 will test this argument.

3 This is known as the theory of the second best.

consumer/physician team will make decisions using net price (net of insurance), but medical care firms will make decisions using gross price. Hence, the slope at a point like S in Fig. 6.3 will not equal the slope of society's production possibility curve. In other words, the reduced price of medical care (because of insurance) will induce the consumption of more medical care than at a Pareto optimal point, given the nonzero insurance elasticity of demand for care (see Chapter 2).[4] We cannot conclude that insurance has necessarily made individuals worse off, however, for the model described in Figs. 6.1 through 6.4 did not take account of uncertainty and individuals' desires to avoid large random losses. Medical insurance provides utility by reducing the risk of large financial losses (see Fig. 2.6), and this utility gain should be balanced against the cost of inducing greater demand for medical care to determine a Pareto optimal point. Of course, if demand were perfectly inelastic (an insurance elasticity of zero), there would be no cost from inducing additional demand. This is why the study of demand is important to the desirable structure of health insurance (see p. 4). The lower the insurance elasticity of demand for the service, the more desirable is coverage, other things equal, because risk is reduced at less cost [3,4,5,6].

A second effect of insurance as presently written was discussed in Chapter 4. There is little or no incentive for insured individuals to search out suppliers that deliver the same product at a lower price. If virtually all individuals in a market are insured, inefficient firms can continue to exist. This type of inefficiency was not even discussed in Figs. 6.1 through 6.4, but can be illustrated by relabeling the isoquants in Fig. 6.1. For example, an efficient firm may produce on the isoquants labeled 1 and 2, but an inefficient firm may require the inputs shown by isoquant 2 to produce an amount of output represented by isoquant 1. In practice, such an inefficiency could cause large losses in community welfare (that is, could cause society to operate well within its utility possibility frontier).

Widespread insurance also implies that the reimbursement of medical care producers could be above competitive levels. In a competitive market the marginal factor of production (i.e., that person or factor that would leave the industry if price were slightly lower) receives a rate of pay reflecting what the factor could earn in its next best alternative. If it were paid a lower rate than the next best alternative, it would leave the industry; if it

---

4 Crew [2] has argued that limitations on entry into medicine induce monopoly rents that make some subsidy optimal. Two observations might be made about this argument: (1) Within Crew's framework the optimal price equals marginal cost. Because marginal cost exceeds zero, the optimal subsidy cannot make the price zero, that is, cannot be complete insurance; (2) The effect of insurance on price competition among suppliers may induce a potentially large distortion, for which Crew does not account. See below.

were paid a higher rate, other factors now in alternative occupations should enter and bid the rate of pay down. (The entering factors are the marginal factors in the alternative occupations.)

Widespread insurance tends to defeat price competition in markets for factors of production. For the same reason that inefficient producers can remain in business (Chapter 4), medical care firms that pay above competitive wages or individual providers who charge above competitive rates can remain in business. Thus, with widespread insurance, medical factors of production (for example, physicians, nurses, aides) could earn above competitive rates of reimbursement; that is, could earn economic rents. At a minimum, such rents, if they exist, transfer income from the rest of the community to producers of medical care. Over time the rents may induce additional entry into the health professions (do the current numbers wanting to attend medical school reflect above competitive returns in medicine?) and distort the fraction of society's resources in medical care.

To summarize this section, a perfectly competitive organization assumes that the consumer's preferences should be honored, an arguable assumption in medical care. Equity does not appear to be an important conceptual objection to competitive organization in medical care. If a competitive organization is adopted, mechanisms need to be found that protect the consumer against large random losses in wealth, while not causing large welfare losses by eliminating the incentive for firms to be efficient in producing services. Such mechanisms will be discussed after a discussion of regulation as a substitute for competitive organization.

REGULATION OR PLANNING OF MEDICAL SERVICES

Present institutions financing medical care could be replaced by public-utility-type regulation or public production of medical care services, as some national health insurance bills propose. An example of a regulated utility is a private airline or the telephone company; an example of public production is a public elementary or secondary school. In either case, a public agency, accountable to the voters, directs resource allocation. (Members of the agency may be appointed by an elected official, as in the case of the Federal Communications Commission, or elected directly, as in the case of a local school board.) The agency's decisions affect what to produce, how to produce, and for whom to produce; in short, the agency answers the questions posed in the opening paragraph of the chapter.

If a similar public agency for medical care were established, the Congress and the agency would determine how much medical care to produce (and thus what is left over for other goods and services) when setting a budget for the medical care sector. The agency would also influence decisions on how to produce; the agency could make decisions itself on questions of how many physicians and how many beds (as the school board decides on how many teachers), or it could adopt rules that heavily influence such decisions (as the Civil Aeronautics Board's rulings on entry and fares affect the number of flights between any two cities). Agency decisions will also influence who gains access to medical services. For example, a decision to ration services using queueing favors those with a low value of time, such as those whose lost time is covered by a sick leave plan, at the expense of those with a high value of time, such as the self-employed. The agency may decide how much the factors of production are paid. For example, the school board sets (or bargains about) teachers' salaries, and the Civil Aeronautics Board's control of fares affects the salaries that airlines can pay.

Placing resource allocation decisions for medical care with a public agency is usually referred to as health planning or a national health service. Sometimes such arrangements are referred to as planning with teeth because past planning efforts have often been cosmetic. Planning with teeth envisions public regulation of a private medical care system; a national health service means public production of medical care services. (The United Kingdom has a national service; Canada has public regulation of a largely private medical care system.)

Health planning is steadily increasing and therefore merits analysis. Although we shall examine planning, much of the discussion also applies to public production.

Let us consider how one prominent approach to national health insurance would resolve the questions posed at the beginning of the chapter.[5] A public agency would determine an overall budget for medical care and the maximum number of hospital beds in a region. Hospitals and physicians would continue to be predominantly private and paid on a fee-for-service basis. If fees exceeded the budgeted amount, all fees would be reduced proportionately. Incentives to produce medical care efficiently would come from the agency's monitoring hospital administrators and medical staffs, attempting to reward good performance with salary increases. (The incentives would be analogous to those given public school administrators to produce education efficiently.) Consumers would be protected against large random losses, because there would be no charges for medical care services. Hence, allocation of medical care among individuals would in principle be based on medical need and would not reflect ability to pay. The total re-

---

5 Specific national health insurance bills are not named because (1) the bills themselves are more complex than the simple description given here; and (2) the bills change over time.

sources in medical care would be decided by the public agency, rather than by the aggregate of individual choices that occurs in a market.

What problems might arise if medical care were organized in this fashion? First, the regulatory process itself consumes resources. Determining budgets and monitoring performance is costly, and any benefits should exceed these costs.[6] Second, demand might exceed the amount an agency would supply. If so, queues or other rationing devices would replace price as a determinant of who receives services. Many argue that the current distribution of income is inequitable, and so should not affect the distribution of medical services. In other words, who receives services should not be based on ability to pay (price). This argument is a form of the equity issue discussed above, and the analysis there applies. In addition, rationing devices other than price could impose a "deadweight" loss; that is, some could be made worse off without making others better off. If you have to stand in line and could have used the time productively, you are worse off and no one else is better off. (I am not considering here the possibility of a temporary queue caused by a random peak in demand.)

Another problem is the possibility for industry capture.[7] What is industry capture? The regulator usually finds it more expensive to obtain information about demand and technology than does the industry. As a result, the regulator frequently begins to rely on the industry for information, and so becomes vulnerable to distortions in the information. Moreover, the industry usually has much more at stake in the agency's decision than any particular member of the general public. Hence, the industry is much more likely than the general public to sue the regulatory agency if the agency's decision is unpalatable. The asymmetric threat of suit may create a pro-industry bias on the part of the regulatory body, a form of capture. Finally, the legislation establishing the agency may charge it with maintaining the industry's "health." In other industries, such a mandate has led to a bias against technological change and protection of existing firms. If new, more efficient technology damages existing firms, the regulatory agency may hinder its introduction.

In addition to these pressures that operate on virtually all regulatory bodies, one force for industry capture occurs when a regulator affects life-and-death decisions. If physicians argue that certain equipment is necessary for saving human lives and can identify human lives that will be saved, the regulatory body will be hard put not to allow installation of the equipment.

---

6 The consumer must monitor performance in either a regulatory or market environment in order to choose a provider. The agency's regulatory role does not relieve the consumer of this burden.

7 See [7] for a general discussion. Evidence is provided in [8] that experience with Certificate of Need legislation is consistent with industry capture.

For example, extension of the Medicare program to those suffering from end-stage renal disease (kidney failure requiring dialysis) was probably guaranteed once it became clear that certain individuals would die without access to dialysis machines [9]. Similarily, expansion of a burn unit is likely if its supporters can point to a certain person's life that would have been saved had new equipment been in place. In such circumstances a regulatory body can say no only with great difficulty.

It could be argued that the optimal action for the regulatory body is approval, that the preferences of individuals in the community are to provide kidney dialysis or expand the burn unit. In any particular case such an argument may be correct. Introduction of a regulatory body, however, changes the decisionmaking process in a subtle way that increases the delivery of services relative to a perfectly competitive market. Individuals who sit on the regulatory body must now take responsibility for identifiable life-and-death decisions, whereas in an impersonal market individuals would not do so.

Consider the case of an air bag in an automobile. Suppose (and this is critical) that individuals are presumed competent to judge whether they wish to forego other goods and services to enjoy the added safety afforded by an air bag. Some may decide they want the air bag; others may decide against it. For concreteness, suppose that half the consumers want the air bag. If all markets are competitive, half of the autos will be produced with air bags; conditional upon the income distribution, that will be the optimal number, as the argument in the first section of the chapter showed. (If you object to this conclusion, place yourself in a world with an optimal income distribution. Would you still object?)

Now suppose that instead of a market there is a regulator of air bags. The regulator must make a decision on the fraction of autos that are to have air bags. Of course, the regulator could decree that half the autos are to have air bags. If this is done, however, some consumer will inevitably be killed or maimed for lack of an air bag. Then the regulator could well be blamed for not decreeing that all autos should have air bags, or may feel guilt at not so decreeing. (Note that the regulator, when making a decision, will not know that half the consumers would have purchased air bags if the decision were left to them, and neither will those who accuse the regulator of making a mistake if air bags are not mandated for all autos.) The desire not to be identified as an individual who made a decision that led to injury gives the regulator an incentive to protect that does not exist in a competitive market.

Because many medical care decisions concern the treatment of illness or injury of identifiable individuals, a medical care sector regulator will probably protect more than a market would. Note, however, that the market outcome is optimal only on the assumption that consumer preferences should be honored.[8] But consumers may recognize their lack of information and wish the regulator to make decisions for them. It might even be argued that any resulting overprotection is a better outcome than the outcome if ill-informed consumers made their own choices.

Suppose there is a drug that helps a certain medical problem but has harmful side effects. Suppose further that if most consumers were well informed, they would not want the drug, although some would. Further suppose that if the drug is marketed, many physicians will prescribe it, and many ill-informed consumers will buy it. It may be better to prohibit marketing of the drug (thus depriving the minority that wanted it) than to allow anyone to purchase it. Similarly, it may be better to force all consumers to purchase autos with air bags than to allow some deaths from motor vehicle accidents. The smaller the minority adversely affected and the more difficult the adverse consequences are to understand without specialized information, the stronger the case for uniform regulation. Overprotection will in some instances lower the amount of resources in medical care (for example, prohibiting drugs), but seems more likely to increase resources because failure to allocate resources can sometimes have adverse consequences that can be traced back to the regulator's decision. Thus for a variety of reasons, the medical care regulator (or public producer) may be captured.

A general problem other than industry capture associated with planning and regulation is its weakening of incentives for efficient production relative to a competitive market. In the competitive market, firms that are not efficient are forced out of business by those that are, because efficient firms can produce the same product at a lower price, and consumers will choose to purchase the lowest-priced product. A regulated firm or a public agency typically does not have the same incentive, because it does not compete with other firms on the basis of price. A public school, for example, does not necessarily lose students if it is inefficient; the inefficiency may simply lead to an increased budget.

In medical care prospective reimbursement is frequently discussed as a substitute for market forces in giving hospitals an incentive for efficiency. If

---

8 Richard Zeckhauser [10] has observed that identification of the individual to be saved leads to more protection. He argues that society has been willing to pay to preserve a myth that no expense should be spared to save a life. If air bags are left to market decisions, society may rationalize the individual's failure to purchase one in a way that preserves the myth. It is more difficult to rationalize the myth with a regulator. Assuming an unregulated outcome does not impair the myth, one cannot say whether the regulator overprotects or the market underprotects. In effect the standard of reference (tastes) has changed; one must decide to satisfy one set of tastes (unidentified lives) or other (identified lives). Zeckhauser also notes that the price of preserving the myth may now be getting so high that we may soon abandon it.

reimbursement is prospective, hospitals receive a budget each year in advance rather than being reimbursed for treatment rendered to individual patients after the fact. Prospective reimbursement appears to give the hospital a budget constraint, just like the perfectly competitive firm in Fig. 6.1. Would the hospital then act like the competitive firm and maximize output for this budget constraint? Unfortunately for the effectiveness of prospective reimbursement, the hospital probably would not. For the outcome to resemble the competitive outcome, the hospital must not be able to influence its budget constraint. Yet it has a clear incentive to do so. The hospital may tell the regulator that hospital services cost $X; the regulator is not well placed to challenge. Put another way, prospective reimbursement differs from the competitive case unless the regulator can monitor the hospital and not reimburse it for inefficient production.

Suppose, for example, that the hospital grants its employees a wage increase above a market level. The regulator must deny such an increase; the regulator's ability to do so, however, especially if denial provokes a strike, is questionable. But suppose the regulator attempts to avoid such a problem by telling the hospital to live within its budget. The hospital might grant the wage increase, exceed the budget the regulator has set for it, and cover its deficit by borrowing. It might then attempt to pay off its loan by artificially inflating its budget the next year. In practice, it is difficult for the regulatory agency to prevent such behavior (except for gross violations) unless it devotes many resources to examining the hospital's inputs and output or else does not make a considered decision of what output may not be produced. For example, giving the hospital a budget increase of 5 percent each year will preclude the production of certain services, but without close examination neither the identity of these services nor whether the community would be willing to pay for them will be known.

An additional problem with planning or regulatory arrangements is their precluding trades in which both parties are made better off *in their own eyes* (see Fig. 6.3). The problem arises because the agency attempts to distribute services among consumers on the basis of medical need rather than demand. For example, suppose I need orthodontic work (teeth straightening) costing $2,000, but would rather have $1,500 in cash. You would be willing to pay $2,000 for cosmetic surgery, but do not need it by the criterion of medical need. If resources are allocated in accordance with need, I get the orthodontia and you get nothing. Suppose, however, I am issued a transferable voucher for $2,000 of medical services instead of being provided with orthodontia. If I sell the voucher to you for $1,750, we are both better off. Because I preferred $1,500 in cash to the orthodontia, I must prefer $1,750 in cash to the orthodontia. You in turn can use the voucher to pay for the cosmetic surgery; however, instead of paying $2,000 for the cosmetic surgery, you will only pay $1,750. Thus, we are both better off, although resources are not allocated on the basis of medical need; allocating resources on the basis of need is not Pareto optimal.

What assumptions lay behind this result? First, it is assumed that other goods or services can substitute for medical care services and leave the consumer equally well off. Thus, there is some amount of money (i.e., other goods and services) that I would accept in lieu of orthodontia and feel equally well off. This assumption is almost certainly true for decisions not having to do with life and death; if I am given other things I value to compensate, I may be able to live with a certain amount of pain or discomfort.

Even in the case of life-and-death decisions, I may prefer to accept money on behalf of my heirs. Suppose, for example, that there is a $100,000 operation that has a 1 in 1,000 chance of extending life for three months. Without the operation, I will die tomorrow. There is a presumptive medical need for the operation, and if resources are allocated in accordance with medical need, I would probably get the operation. But given the small likelihood of success and the small extension of life, I might rather see the $100,000 given to my children or to charity and forgo the operation.

Second, the consumer is assumed to know what is best. If I trade orthodontia for $1,750 in cash, I am presumed to be making an informed choice. If I don't know that failure to obtain the orthodontic services could lead in a few years to the inability to chew food, there is no presumption that I am making a desirable choice.

Third, the income distribution is assumed to be acceptable. If I am poor, but you are rich, society may not permit us to trade. However, even if the income distribution is not acceptable, it is still true that both of us can be made better off without making someone else worse off if we can trade. Moreover, the fundamental theorem of welfare economics implies that the proper remedy for an objectionable income distribution is redistribution of cash income rather than redistribution in kind (e.g., medical services for the poor), provided that consumers are presumed to be the best judge of their own welfare.[9] Redistribution in cash allows the consumer to select any point along the budget line, whereas redistribution in kind will in general preclude attaining the highest possible indifference curve.

---

9 Although the discussion has stressed the consumer's ignorance as a reason why one may conclude that the consumer is not the best judge of the consumer's welfare, a different argument for subsidizing medical care for the poor is that the "donor" (taxpayer) receives utility from the way in which the poor spend the money that is being redistributed. This argument accepts the optimality of the prior income distribution, but argues that the middle class wishes to make transfers to the poor of specific services as well as generalized purchasing power. The resolution of questions having to do with the amount and form of transfers must take place through the political process.

Thus, if consumers are the best judge of their own welfare, the case for public utility regulation is weakened. But even if the consumer is conceded to be less than well informed, it does not follow that regulation is an appropriate remedy for two reasons. First, consumers are as ignorant in their voting role as in their consuming role and will exert influence over a regulatory agency in their role as voters [10].[10] One example showing the influence of consumers even with regulation is the recent controversy over saccharin (an artificial sweetener). The Food and Drug Administration wished to ban saccharin because when taken in large doses, it causes cancer in animals. The public outcry over the proposed ban was sufficiently strong that the Congress delayed implementing the ban for eighteen months pending further study. Although the Food and Drug Administration argued that an informed consumer would not choose to eat saccharin,[11] the tastes of the "ignorant" consumers of saccharin nevertheless prevailed, at least for the moment. Thus, regulation in the context of a democratic political process cannot necessarily overcome presumptively ignorant consumers' tastes.

Second, the regulator also lacks critical information. While the regulator can learn relatively easily about the technical possibilities (for example, can learn that a particular operation has a 1 in 1,000 chance of success), it is very difficult for the regulator to learn the consumer's preferences. In the previous chapter I argued that much of the marginal unit of medical care produced intangibles. Intangibles such as relief of anxiety and heroic efforts near the end of life are likely to be valued differently by different individuals. I may be willing to spend $15 to see if my sore throat is serious; given the odds that it is not serious, you may prefer to use the money for other purposes. I may be willing to spend $12,000 for a coronary bypass graft operation that relieves pain from angina pectoris; you may rather have the $12,000 for something else. I may want heroic efforts taken near the end of life with their associated costs; you may want to leave the money to heirs.

The regulator is likely to make uniform decisions that lead us both to take the same action. If visits to the physician are free, we will both go for our sore throat, even though you would have rather had the $15 in cash that the physician was paid. If coronary bypass operations are not provided, I would have been willing to pay the cost of getting one. In a nutshell, the

10 The differences are that votes are not weighted by the distribution of wealth and that specific preferences are quite difficult to transmit through the political process because voting for candidates usually takes place along several dimensions at once (which makes a random outcome more likely).

11 Although the Food and Drug Administration's decision was based on a law that substances shown to cause cancer in animals must be prohibited, a number of its public pronouncements effectively made the point that an informed consumer would not eat saccharin.

planner is relatively well placed to know the technical possibilities, but poorly placed to know how those possibilities are valued; the consumer has the opposite problem. Although it is obvious that the consumer's knowledge is not that of the health professional's and so the outcome of market processes in medical care may not resemble the outcome if consumers were well informed, regulation or planning does not necessarily improve the outcome. In fact, neither the consumer nor the regulator is omniscient.

CHANGING MEDICAL CARE INSTITUTIONS TO MORE CLOSELY RESEMBLE A COMPETITIVE MARKET

Suppose we took the view that a market-like organization was desirable. Such a view implies the consequences of consumer ignorance are for the most part tolerable; for many decisions consumers would be free to make their own mistakes. A market-like organization also implies the income distribution is acceptable; however, if the current distribution is not acceptable, it can be altered by changing the existing tax and transfer programs (tax reform and welfare reform).

If a market-like organization of medical care were to be instituted, how would medical care be organized? One possibility is that health insurance policies would contain substantial deductibles. The deductible would be large enough that most of the population, most of the time, would not exceed it. In that case most consumers would not be subsidized and so would not increase their demand for medical care above the level in a competitive market. The population would be left bearing some risk (as discussed in Chapter 2), but if the deductible is not overly large (or is related to income), the amount of risk would not be very large.[12]

For the half of medical care services rendered outside the hospital, such a deductible will probably bring about a market organization while protecting against risk. A problem will remain for hospital and inpatient physician services, however. Although most of the population, most of the time, does not exceed the deductible, the marginal dollar for most hospitalized patients must be heavily subsidized if the population is to be protected against large losses in wealth. In this case the market for hospital and inpatient physician services tends to break down, as described in Chapter 4. Thus, even with a moderately large deductible, today's "basic" health insurance or "major medical" health insurance will inhibit a market organization for hospital and inpatient physician services.

Fortunately, other possibilities for introducing market-like organization also leave the consumer protected against large losses in wealth. These possibilities vary the insured's premium depending on the particular provider or

---

12 For empirical support for this statement, see [12].

hospital chosen. There are two existing methods for varying the premium. One is so-called indemnity insurance. An indemnity insurance policy pays a certain amount of dollars per unit of services consumed, for example, $100 per hospital day or $8 per office visit. The premium for the policy increases as the dollars paid per unit of service increase.

Such insurance may pay much of the consumer's bill (thereby averting the possibility of large losses), but the consumer who uses the more expensive hospital or physician will bear the entire marginal cost of doing so. Such insurance at least lays a basic for price competition among providers of medical care services. Hospital admission and length of stay decisions (quantity decisions) are still made using subsidized prices (potentially causing the distortions described above), but the large increases in hospital expenditures have not resulted from increases in the number of patient days, but rather rapidly increasing cost per patient day. Table 6.1 shows the rate of increase in these two components from 1950 to 1973; the annual rate of percentage increase has been 1.2 percent for patient days, but 9.1 percent for expense per patient day. Thus, much of the probable distortion in the use of resources induced by present insurance arrangements could be addressed by the use of indemnity insurance.

The benefits of indemnity insurance will be reduced to the degree that the consumer has difficulty obtaining information or faces constrained choices. The consumer may be unable to ascertain how much a hospital stay is likely to cost at alternative hospitals, and the consumer's choices among hospitals are restricted by the physician's staff privileges (the patient must go to hospitals where the physician can admit patients). Under such circumstances the outcome may well differ from that observed in a market of well-informed consumers.

Table 6.1 Components of hospital expenditure

Year	Patient days per 1,000 people	Expense per patient day*	Admissions per 1,000 people	Expense per admission*
1950	900.5	$ 15.62	110.5	$127.23
1960	980.0	32.23	128.9	244.54
1970	1197.9	81.01	145.0	668.67
1973	1194.5	114.69	152.6	897.20
Average annual percentage increase 1950–1973				
	1.2	9.1	1.4	8.9

Source: Social Security Administration, "Medical Care Expenditures, Prices, and Costs. Background Book" (DHEW Publication No. (SSA) 75-11909), pp. 34, 37.

*Part of the increase in later years is attributable to increased expenses for outpatient departments. However, accounting for outpatient expenses would change these figures only negligibly; see the adjusted expenses in the source.

Another relatively well-known alternative to existing arrangements is prepaid group practice.[13] Prepaid group practices are groups of physicians that may operate their own hospital, but in any event agree to supply medical care in return for a fixed periodic premium. To attract patients, the group's monthly premium cannot be out of line with the price charged for medical care from alternative sources. Thus, there can be price competition among providers. Care may be rationed among subscribers to the prepaid group practice on grounds other than money price, but the consumer is presumtively aware of any such rationing when selecting prepaid group practice or when renewing membership in one already used.

Unfortunately, prepaid group practices are not now very significant in the medical marketplace, enrolling only 2 percent of the population [13].[14] Their growth has been slow for several reasons. They are difficult to organize. Second, most persons obtain medical insurance through their place of employment. Unless employers offer the prepaid group as an option, the group competes at a severe disadvantage. Even when offered as an option, a prepaid group may find it difficult to attract physicians who have already established practices. (Patients of established physicians may not be able to elect prepaid group practice through their employer-provided insurance.) If physician recruiting must be limited to new graduates, the group will have difficulty accommodating rapid growth.

Recently, public policy has attempted to assist prepaid group practices. If the group practice can become certified and is accepting new patients, large employers in an area must offer it as an option to their employees. Unfortunately, to become certified requires delivering a sufficiently diverse number of medical services that the certified group practices may not be competitive; as a result, there are few groups certified [14]. (Recent amendments to the law have addressed this issue.) Another source of assistance is the substantial increase in new physicians fostered by public policy for other reasons (see Chapter 3). Greater numbers of new physicians should make it easier for prepaid group practices to recruit physicians. Nevertheless, it would take an extreme optimist to believe that prepaid group practices will achieve a predominant share of the market any time soon.

Two other possibilities for introducing market-like incentives into the hospital sector have not been tried yet, but do not appear to have the disad-

---

13 Prepaid group practices are sometimes known as Health Maintenance Organizations (HMOs). However, the term HMO is also used to refer to a group of physicians that may encompass all physicians in a county or local market area, thereby precluding price competition. I therefore use the term prepaid group practice.

14 In some localities (principally on the West Coast), however, their market share is approximately 20 percent.

vantages of indemnity insurance and prepaid group practices. The first is Variable Cost Insurance (VCI [15, 16, 17]), which has analogies with indemnity insurance. Although it could cover physician services, VCI is designed principally for hospital services. Under VCI each hospital in an area would receive an expense rating. The rating would be proportional to the unit price of treating cases at that hospital. The insured would choose a hospital or set of hospitals and would pay a premium proportional to the rating of the hospital chosen. If the insured goes to a different hospital than the one chosen, the policy pays what would have been paid at the hospital chosen. Analytically this arrangement is similar to indemnity insurance, except the consumer has better information about the costliness of alternative hospitals when choosing the amount of the indemnity. The better information might also cause some physicians to modify their pattern of staff privileges.

The second untried alternative has analogies with prepaid group practice and is termed the Health Care Alliance [18]. The Alliance idea attempts to sidestep the problems of establishing new prepaid groups or expanding existing groups. An insurance company can form an Alliance by designating a group of physicians for which it specifies a premium. A consumer's eligibility for that premium is contingent on using physicians in the Alliance (or physicians to whom they refer patients). The premium for the Alliance is proportional to expenses generated by the physicians in the Alliance. Thus, physicians who hospitalize frequently, use expensive hospitals, frequently bring in consulting physicians, or charge high fees will have high expense ratings. Alliances can compete with other Alliances partially on the basis of price.

The Alliance idea and prepaid group practice have more potential for salutary effects than indemnity insurance or Variable Cost Insurance because they are more comprehensive. They provide incentives not to hospitalize in marginal cases and in general apply to the quantity of services demanded, whereas the other methods do not. Unfortunately, there is also a possible problem with both prepaid group practices and the Alliance idea. If premiums are set straightforwardly on the basis of the expense the physician generates, it is in the interests of the physician not to treat expensive or sickly patients. (This problem does not apply to VCI or indemnity insurance because they operate only on unit price, not on total expense.) Although it can be mandated that groups or Alliances accept patients on a nondiscriminatory basis (so-called open enrollment), the incentive remains for the group to persuade sickly patients to seek care elsewhere (through a discourteous manner, long waits, and the like). If the provider's premium were adjusted for the sickliness of the patients treated so that any differences among provider groups reflected solely differences in how similar groups of patients were treated, sickly patients would not face a potential access problem. Unfortunately, no satisfactory methodology for making such an adjustment exists at present; the payoff from finding one, however, is reason to experiment with the Alliance concept.

We have delineated three different ways to finance or organize medical care services.[15] The first is the status quo—nearly complete insurance for hospitals and steadily more complete insurance of non-hospital services. Such insurance increases demand for medical care and greatly reduces or eliminates the basis for price competition, but does not cause any access problems and protects consumers against large random losses in wealth from illness. It may, however, lead to more resources in medical care than society wishes, inefficient production and (possibly) above competitive rates of renumeration for medical care factors of production.

The second is a planning or regulatory approach (or possibly public production). If consumers find it sufficiently difficult to become informed, they may wish a regulator to make choices for them. Rationing of services would be on a basis other than price and so consumers would be protected against large random losses in wealth. The problems of such an approach include possible capture by the industry, weaker incentives for efficient production than in a market with price competition, and the planner's inability to know the consumer's preferences. Such an approach need not pose access problems for sickly patients; however, it may pose access problems for others. If, for example, waiting time is used to ration services, those with high values of time will be discouraged and there will be a deadweight loss for all who use services. The regulatory process itself is costly; not only must the regulator's salary be paid (and costs paid to generate the information needed), but legal challenges to the regulator may also be costly to litigate.

A third way to finance medical care is to reintroduce marketplace incentives, specifically price competition. Marketplace incentives can lead to producing efficiently the amount of medical care that consumers demand. Certain mechanisms for introducing price competition into the hospital sector may pose access problems (but that is not known).

In the end consumers must decide through the political process whether they feel sufficiently well informed to make choices individually, whether they would rather delegate choice to a planner, or whether they prefer the known distortions of the status quo. In light of the persistent calls for reforming medical care financing, the choice appears to be between the plan and the market alternatives.

REFERENCES

1. Francis M. Bator. "The Simple Analytics of Welfare Maximization." *American Economic Review* 47, No. 1: 22–59 (March 1957).

2. Michael Crew. "Coinsurance and the Welfare Economics of Medical Care." *American Economic Review* 59, No. 5: 906–908 (December 1969).

3. Martin S. Feldstein. "The Welfare Loss of Excess Health Insurance." *Journal of Political Economy* 81, No. 2: 251–280 (March–April 1973).

4. John M. Marshall. "Moral Hazard." *American Economic Review* 66, No. 5: 880–890 (December 1976)

5. Mark V. Pauly. "The Economics of Moral Hazard: Comment." *American Economic Review* 58, No. 3: 531–537 (June 1968).

6. Richard J. Zeckhauser. "Medical Insurance: A Case Study of the Tradeoff Between Risk Spreading and Appropriate Incentives." *Journal of Economic Theory* 2, No. 1: 10–26 (March 1970).

7. Roger G. Noll. "The Consequences of Public Utility Regulation of Hospitals." In *Controls on Health Care*, edited by Ruth Hanft and Paul Rettig. Washington: National Academy of Sciences, 1975.

8. David S. Salkever and Thomas W. Bice. "The Impact of Certificate-of-Need Controls on Hospital Investment." *Milbank Memorial Fund Quarterly/Health and Society* 54, No. 2: 185–214 (Spring 1976).

9. Richard Zeckhauser. "Procedures for Valuing Lives. *Public Policy* 23, No. 4: 419–464 (Fall 1975).

10. Richard J. Zeckhauser. "Coverage for Catastrophic Illness." *Public Policy* 21, No. 2: 149–172 (Spring 1973).

11. Mark V. Pauly. "Is Medical Care Different?" Paper given at a Federal Trade Commission Conference on Competition in the Health Care Sector: Past, Present, and Future. Washington, D.C.: (June 1977).

12. Emmett B. Keeler, Daniel Morrow, and Joseph P. Newhouse. "The Demand for Supplementary Health Insurance, or Do Deductibles Matter? *Journal of Political Economy* 85, No. 4: 789–802 (August 1977).

13. Lawrence Goldberg and Warren Greenberg. "The Health Maintenance Organization and Its Effects on Competition." Federal Trade Commission, Bureau of Economics, (July 1977).

14. Paul Starr. "The Undelivered Health System." *The Public Interest* 42: 66–85 (Winter 1976).

15. Joseph P. Newhouse and Vincent Taylor. "How Shall We Pay for Hospital Care?" *The Public Interest* 23: 78–92 (Spring 1971).

16. Joseph P. Newhouse and Vincent Taylor. "The Subsidy Problem in Hospital Insurance." *Journal of Business* 43, No. 4: 452–456 (October 1970).

17. Joseph P. Newhouse and Vincent Taylor. "A New Type of Hospital Insurance." *The Journal of Risk and Insurance* 38: 601–612 (December 1971).

18. Paul M. Ellwood and Walter McClure. "Health Delivery Reform." Mimeo, 1976 (available from InterStudy, Excelsior, Minnesota).

19. Alain C. Enthoven and Roger G. Noll. "Regulatory and Nonregulatory Strategies for Controlling Health Care Costs." Stanford University Graduate School of Business, Research Paper No. 402.

Index

Adverse selection, 21-22, 111-112

Biomedical research, 81-82
Budget line, 5-6, 37

Canadian national health insurance,
   17, 18, 57-58, 101
Certificate of Need legislation, 72
Consumer ignorance, 54-55, 97-98
Contract curve, 91
Cost containment regulation, 72

Deductible, 12-14, 17-18, 20, 108
Demand for health insurance, 19-23
Demand for medical care
   empirical estimates, 15-19
   physician demand creation, 55-61
   theory, 4-15

Efficiency, 90
Employment in medical care, 1
Entry restriction, 53-54
Equity, 95-97, 102
Expansion path, 37
Expenditure for medical care
   different countries compared, 85-
     87

Fallacy of composition, 63-64

Health Care Alliances, 111-112
Health insurance
   demand for, 19-23
   and price competition, 61-65
Health planning, 32-47, 100-108
Hospitals, economic theory of, 68-73

Income effect, 7-8
Indemnity insurance, 109
Index number problem, 76n
Indifference curves, 5-6, 93-94
Industry capture, 102-104
Infant mortality, 78-79
Isoquant, 36-39, 90-92

Joint cost, 29-33

Manpower planning, 32-47
Medical marketplace
   divergences from perfect competi-
     tion, 50-65
Medical need, 105-106
Medical schools
   enrollment, 27, 32-47
   federal policy toward, 25-27
   financing, 26-32

Morbidity, 77-78, 83-84
Mortality, 75-76, 79-81

Nonprofit firm, theory of, 68-73
Normative economics, definition, 41-
    42

Occam's Razor, 61

Pareto optimality, 90-100, 105-106
Physicians
    hours of work, 50-53
    numbers to train, 45-47
Physiological measures of health, 82-
    83
Positive economics, definition, 41-42
Post hoc ergo propter hoc fallacy, 77
Prepaid group practice, 110
Price competition, 61-65, 99-100
Price discrimination, 96-97

Prices in medical care, 2
Production function, 38-39, 75
Production function estimation, 39-41
Production possibility curve, 91-92, 94
Prospective reimbursement, 104-105
Pure cost, 29-33

Regulation, 100-108
Rent, 53-54, 99-100
Risk aversion, 19-20, 98-99

Second best, 98
Substitution effect, 7-8, 14

Time cost, 11, 102

Usual, customary, and reasonable, 64
Utility-possibility frontier, 94-95, 99

Variable Cost Insurance, 111